Move, F[...] Recover

A Workbook

Your Practical Guide to Balancing Mind and Body

Erin Taylor

Illustrations by Rebekah MacKay

VELO press

Ironman® is a registered trademark of World Triathlon Corporation

Published by:

an imprint of Ulysses Press
PO Box 3440
Berkeley, CA 94703
www.velopress.com

VeloPress is the leading publisher of books on sports for passionate and dedicated athletes around the world. Focused on cycling, triathlon, running, swimming, nutrition/diet, and more, VeloPress books help you achieve your goals and reach the top of your game.

ISBN: 978-1-64604-775-8

Printed in the United States
10 9 8 7 6 5 4 3 2 1

Project managers: Brian McLendon, Kierra Sondereker
Managing editor: Claire Chun
Editors: Renee Jardine, Susan Lang
Proofreader: Beret Olsen
Front cover design: Kyle Keigan

Please Note: This book has been written and published strictly for informational purposes, and in no way should be used as a substitute for consultation with health care professionals. You should not consider educational material herein to be the practice of medicine or to replace consultation with a physician or other medical practitioner. The author and publisher are providing you with information in this work so that you can have the knowledge and can choose, at your own risk, to act on that knowledge. The author and publisher also urge all readers to be aware of their health status and to consult health care professionals before beginning any health program.

Move, Rest, Recover

A Workbook

This book is for you.

In memory of Gary Wong.

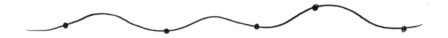

Contents

A Practice for All of Us

Everyone is so busy, doing so much. *When do you rest?*

Recovery is one of the most powerful and accessible tools to support well-being, longevity, and the balance that we are designed for. And yet, it remains one of the most underutilized practices that is available to us—an important opportunity is being missed. I've been teaching yoga for two decades, coaching everyone from Olympians to office workers, and over the years the most startling imbalance I see is between working and resting. It's everywhere I look:

My friend whose schedule makes my head spin just hearing about their back-to-back weekend activities…

Competitive athletes who turn up to stretch out and can't seem to shift the muscle memory of training at full speed…

The many moms I've worked with, with children ranging from a few months old to well into their teens, who struggle to set down the all-encompassing load of motherhood…

People in my community whose only accessible yoga session of the week is so often displaced by the relentless and boundary-less demands of work and life load…

I've written this book for all of us.

When I first started teaching, I was fortunate to have the opportunity to use my experience and skills to support collegiate athletes. As a former university basketball player, I was well-versed in the demands and rhythms of competing at that level and had begun developing an approach to use yoga in a sports context. It was less about being able to put your foot behind your head and more about developing the knowledge and understanding of how what you do on the mat benefits you on the track, trail, court, field, lake, river, and beyond.

I'd show up with all kinds of ideas about what we might do to ease the sport-specific imbalances spread across the stadium concourse where I met different teams to practice. And while I could clearly see hamstrings overburdened by dysfunctional glutes, locked hips due to constant stopping and pivoting, and severely internally rotated shoulders from hours of swinging rackets, I nearly always had to drop my agenda and focus on the starkest imbalance of all—these young women and men were desperate for rest.

It's not just about doing yoga, it's how you use it that matters.

While they needed to activate and strengthen their upper back, core, and glutes, to access more fluidity in their bodies, and to move in more nonhabitual ways to maintain biomechanical balance, these actions became the subtext of our time together. What was more urgent was the need to slow down and meet themselves where they were—to become aware of imbalance, and to respond accordingly. So that's what we did. Sure, we stretched and realigned, but the main focus of our practice was to rest and recover.

This approach isn't just effective for athletes. I've witnessed the benefits of restorative practice over many years, across many different contexts, and its unique ability to create an internal reconnecting of the dots. The results are undeniable: recovery works. You just have to practice.

Rest works.

I encourage people to practice a little, often, until we next meet. A week passes, sometimes more. Most admit they haven't done anything since the last class, and now they say they really need a reset. Why is that? It's something I think about daily: What moves someone to practice? What stops us from starting, and from staying with it? Too often, we wait to rest until that decision is made for us—when we're sidelined by injury, signed off sick, or stuck in a deep valley of fatigue. But we don't have to.

Don't worry, I'm not here to police your practice. I get it. I feel like resting is part of my job, and yet I forget how and when to use it all the time. It's a forever practice. Recovery is just as important as everything else that we do, and it's time that we recognize this simple truth and honor it as reality.

While your restorative journey is unique and personal, I hope your time here inspires you to make rest yours and to create a practice that truly supports you, wherever you are.

Erin

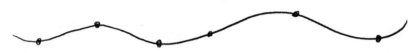

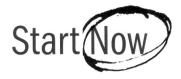

Start Now

Hello and welcome to your recovery practice. Well done for being here!

Put your feet up and make yourself comfortable. It's okay; this is just as important as everything else that you do. Not that you need permission to pause.

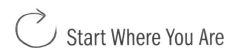

Start Where You Are

Yes, right here, right now. Just begin.

- Sit comfortably and close your eyes.
- Take a deep breath in… a slow breath out…
- Continue to deepen your breathing.
- Notice your breath slow and steady, and focus on the sensations of your breath moving in and out through your nose while you allow the expression on your face to soften.
- Continue for 5 more deep breaths.
- Open your eyes.
- Pause and feel the difference.

Guess what? You've just activated recovery. That's right—you can recharge momentarily and clear the chaos in an instant. Transitioning from work to relaxation, from effort to ease, and refueling yourself in the moments when you need it the most doesn't require anything fancy. You don't need any gadgets, a completely crossed-off to-do list, or a picture-perfect studio. No grand gesture required. All you need to harness the power of real recovery is your attention.

> This is less about self-improvement and more about meeting yourself and being well where you are.

Create Your Recovery Practice

There's so much science affirming the importance of rest and so many tools available to support us and yet, *do you feel rested? Well, do you?* There's an abundance of research telling us we're overdoing in life and ever-increasing resources at the ready to help us recharge, and yet recovery remains one of the most underutilized tools available to us. This book isn't a science project, nor is it a quick performance fix or life hack—it's a tool to connect you to rest, and to equip you with the knowledge and understanding to act on it in a meaningful way.

This requires deep reflection on your rest—how you are or aren't showing up for recovery and the outcome of your behavior—and a willingness to pause and reflect, and ultimately to create your recovery practice. This is a must-have for thriving in the modern world.

Take a deep breath in...
a slow breath out...
Continue to deepen your breathing.

Keep reading to discover how to tune into your mental and physical state, to more clearly discern what's needed, and to respond with effective practices. Together we will answer these questions:

Why should I rest and recover?

How do I know when to stop and rest?

When I stop, what should I do?

You will find that restorative practice naturally flows into real life and is most powerful when it is fluid enough to honor the practicalities of your moments and days. The best part is that it's right here waiting for you. Yes, now! Practicing in this way connects the dots of your well-being and longevity. It brings you into balance, again and again. You don't have to wait any longer to rest, recover, and feel the difference.

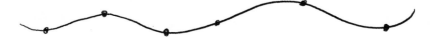

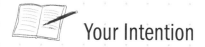

Your Intention

Take a moment now to identify what's brought you here. Consider your intention and write it down!

Why have you opened this book? What do you hope to gain? Don't think too hard, just see what's here—this is your intuition nudging you into action. Note what comes up and revisit these insights as you move forward into your recovery practice.

Use This Book to Catch Your Breath

This space is designed to unwind fatigue and to equip you with the self-awareness, knowledge, and understanding needed to become more fluent in rest. I'll guide you through your restorative journey and help you articulate how to use recovery to full advantage so that you can move through each day more effectively and with more ease.

Together we'll create a restorative foundation that you can lean into whenever you need to shift your perspective and catch your breath. A clear baseline for why recovery matters and how it works, along with practical examples and accessible mental and physical tools, will encourage motivation and momentum in your practice, increase your capacity for meaningful recovery, and make it count.

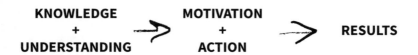

KNOWLEDGE + UNDERSTANDING → **MOTIVATION + ACTION** → **RESULTS**

Commit to the Journey

Use this book as your companion, like a trusted friend, teammate, or coach, to serve your movement, rest, and recovery. Together, we'll explore how to:

 Understand Recovery—Cultivate a Restorative Mindset

 Activate Recovery—Learn to Use Rest

 Strengthen Recovery—Create Your Recovery Practice

Throughout this book you will find these practical, interactive tools to support your rest fluency:

 Recovery Myth: Become aware of myths that keep you from fully recharging and common excuses and misinformation that lead you to put off rest.

 Reflect + Connect: Get your head in the (recovery) game by unpacking and reframing your attitudes and behaviors around rest. Use these prompts to get clear about how you are, what you need, and how to move into real recovery.

 Practice: Move through your days well supported by practical mental and physical rest routines.

Rest Tip: Benefit from easy ways to boost your resets—use these insights to support more effective rest.

 Notice: Use brief checkpoints to prompt meaningful observation in the moment.

 Rest Plan: Make space to plan, track, and review your practice. Use these pages to anchor your wins and keep going!

By the end of this journey, you'll be equipped to harness recovery's superpowers, not only to support yourself, but to help others too.

Make Rest Yours

Your rest is yours. It's a nonlinear and uniquely personal practice. While there is no universal prescription that suits everyone, it's my hope that in the pages ahead you'll catch your breath while gleaning real inspiration and practical new ways to stay buoyant in the moments when you need it most.

Know this: if recovery doesn't fit in your real life, it won't work. Recovery can be a game changer, but the dots have to connect. It's not a sideshow, lip service, or a sporadic massage. You can't just tick the box by closing your eyes and setting a timer, lying on the sofa, or going to a random yoga class. If you value the longevity of your well-being, make rest a main event throughout your day, every day, in your way.

Rest for your real life.

Even if you have a lot going on (who doesn't?), now is the time to disrupt the inertia of doing and access the rest and recovery that we all so urgently need—in the time that you have. When you contextualize recovery based on your unique circumstances and goals, you unlock its power, and by mastering your rest, you'll be in a much better, more balanced state of being. When applied this way, rest is a resilience-boosting superpower, which is why practicality is the connective tissue of your journey to establish your restorative practice.

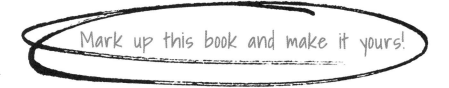
Mark up this book and make it yours!

Your practice is incredibly personal and up to you. Here are a few possibilities of how you can go forward:

- **Full send:** Move through the book sequentially for a comprehensive understanding of how to create and use your recovery practice.

- **In the moment:** Use the table of contents and Practice Now (page 189) to connect to timely practices. A 2-Minute Reset (page 147), anyone?

- **Oracle:** Open to random pages, oracle-style, when you find yourself flagging and needing a bit of inspiration.

Scan the QR code for exclusive *Move, Rest, Recover* audio and video practices, glimpses behind the scenes, guest interviews, and additional resources for your rest and recovery.

Practice and feel the difference.

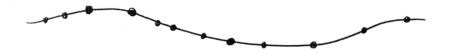

UNDERSTAND RECOVERY

Cultivate a Restorative Mindset

Our days are fully loaded. Work, training, social commitments, life admin, communications… It's an endless conveyor belt of deadlines, health and fitness maintenance, and domestic duties, not to mention emails, texts, and social media to keep up with. Everything is open online, all the time, encouraging us to engage constantly, thanks to an abundance of digital technology that demands our continual productivity and connectivity. We've become fully climatized to always being on, and just thinking about this—and trying to figure out how to rest more—feels difficult, doesn't it?

In a world that is addicted to doing, rest is a brave and progressive movement in the opposite direction.

> Recovery is a rejuvenating internal movement to balance your external action, a recalibration that brings your mind, body, and nervous system into harmony.

It's a Balance

We shape our experience of each day by how we direct our attention and with it, our thoughts and actions. Where our attention goes, our energy flows. Consciously, or more often unconsciously, we are either moving toward balance or away from it. This is as true for harmonizing work and rest as it is for balancing strength and flexibility. When this balance feels most elusive is the time to remember there's no need to be rigid or to constantly weigh one thing against another. You don't have to struggle against the juggle. Perfect balance doesn't exist. Every day is different; there is a natural ebb and flow and, like most aspects of life, recovery is a practice of moving toward balance.

It's no surprise that paying attention to your innate need for balance in a culture that embodies disequilibrium can feel counterintuitive, or even radical. This might cause a small brain explosion (stay with me), but I'll venture to say that rest is the ultimate power stance—it's an inertia-breaking way to value and uphold your well-being. Recovery is a dynamic movement that supports you to more easefully navigate and harmonize your full days in a sustainable way. You might have forgotten you can move toward center daily. How does that work? Balance is a personal practice, and by connecting the dots you'll discover your unique, everyday way.

 Have you considered balance and how rest relates? How are your choices moving you toward balance or away from it?

Balance is a practice.

For All of Us

We can't really start to recover in a meaningful way without first addressing our mindset, which is informed by past experiences and related conditioning, societal pressures, socioeconomic conditions, and myths and misinformation—all of which too often present an array of severe and unjust everyday realities that limit access to rest.

Rest shouldn't be a privilege and yet, too often, it is. The fact is, rest is not a luxury. It's a human necessity that everyone should be able to access, regardless of circumstances like means, time, or space. It's not something to be inherited or earned. And, thankfully, there are unpretentious entry points we can create to this basic life support for ourselves even when we are at our most overworked and undersupported. This is what we're here to explore and practice.

 ## A Momentary Recharge

Okay, let's take a quick break (again, yes) and recharge for a moment to keep us going.

- Close your eyes.
- Gently part your lips and soften your jaw.

- Take 3 deep breaths—slow and steady.
- Open your eyes, keeping your gaze soft, and turn up the corners of your mouth.
- Pause and feel the difference.

Well done. Onward.

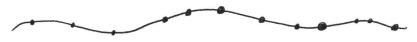

Why should I rest and recover?

Recovery Is Important

Listen, the recovery process is complex and dynamic. If it were easy, you probably wouldn't have opened this book. And it's also quite simple—rest is really important. Recovery is just as important as everything else you do. Pause and let that land for a moment…

Recovery is just as important as everything else you do.

Fatigue significantly impacts cognitive abilities, causing everything from the frustration of needing more time for a simple task, to the severe danger of falling asleep behind the wheel. Tiredness lowers mood and negatively affects mental state and, when left unaddressed, can increase the risk of mental health challenges, such as anxiety and depression.

Your body cannot rebound and grow stronger when your tissues don't have ample time to repair. And your overall energy is a limited yet renewable resource that must be replenished through nutrition and restorative activities.

In the same way that life load and stress can overwhelm your systems and wear you out, rest can fill you up. Rest is, literally, fuel.

 How might rest equip you to…
…absorb the benefits and gains of all your efforts?

…avoid illness, injury, and burnout; to recharge for your next output?

…embody your resilience?

Recovery Is Active

While you might assume that recovery happens by default when you push back from your desk, have that post-run shower, or sip a glass of wine on a Friday night, rejuvenation is not automatic. If you ever struggle to ease the tension of a hard effort, lie awake at night with a busy mind, or still feel a frazzled undercurrent even after a weekend away from work, you know what I'm talking about. Stopping work doesn't mean you're not working. Recovery isn't as straightforward as slipping between the sheets.

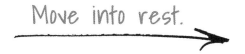

Recovery practice is not a passive substitute for your active practices—your work day, your workout, your parenting, and all the action in between. The input of rest is meant to work in balance with the output of action to move you forward. At the risk of glorifying recovery as yet another way to fuel the endless pursuit of productivity, it is actually a rich and dynamic process that, when done right, works like a superpower to help you feel and perform better. Rest is an intentional movement, a progressive action!

In today's world, we habitually do things so hard and fast, and at such high volume, that many of us find it difficult to access a slower gear. Life's demands too often overshadow our own basic needs, care, and well-being. We're skilled in accelerating from 0 to 60, but find it a lot harder to move in the other direction because we don't do it often enough. Slowing down has become surprisingly unfamiliar and often uncomfortable. It's not that we can't do it, we're just out of practice.

If you value your well-being and longevity, you have to activate and strengthen rest and recovery, on purpose, just as you would train a muscle.

We'll explore how to activate meaningful rest in Activate Recovery (page 57), and how to strengthen your restorative practice with repetition in Strengthen Recovery (page 107).

Recovery Is Readily Available

Thankfully, as you've seen in the two brief practices you've already tried, you don't need any fancy kit, a class, or loads of time to recharge. Restoration shouldn't be relegated to the massage table, bath, or yoga mat. Rest and recovery can and should happen within and alongside life's messy moments (see Rest in the Mess, page 23). As little as 30 seconds can be a game changer (see I Don't Have Time, page 24).

All you need is your attention, your most valuable tool, to access the awareness and response needed to recover in a meaningful way. Momentary gestures, such as looking up from your laptop and feeling your gaze soften, or taking a few deep breaths and allowing your shoulders to drop, can be rejuvenating when you simply notice. Using your attention and self-awareness, you can more clearly discern when it's time to rest and respond with a reset that addresses practicalities, such as your current location or available time.

Rest in the Mess

The next time you feel chaos making demands of you, try flexing your recovery muscle first. Remember that rest can happen even in the mess—pausing to stretch next to the pile of dirty dishes, stepping back from your messy desk, breathing deeply while commuting home from school with your rowdy kids. Choose to slow down, breathe deeply, and pay attention, and you can find rest right in front of you.

 What's a recurring messy moment that you could relax into?

Calm is available, even in the chaos.

I Don't Have Time

Good news! Rest isn't another task to fit in, nor is it something to do for productivity's sake. Phew. Can you feel the collective relief? You can recover in the time that you do have, whether it's 5, 20, or 60 minutes. Just 30 seconds? Great, let's rest! Even brief recharges add up to more ease and better energy.

It's time to ditch the self-defeating mentality that recovery doesn't work, matter, or count without a bigger, more official container of time or place of significance. Rather than skipping recovery because you're time-poor, remember that anything is better than nothing, and the more you practice rest, the more adept you become at recovering efficiently and effectively.

If you wait until everything is done to allow yourself to rest, there won't be any time left. "I can't rest until I do x, y, z..." Sound familiar? This is flawed thinking because it implies that it's not okay to take a break until all tasks are complete and everything is in order, a problematic mentality that you can solve by getting out of your own way. And sure, it all might seem so important. Everything you're doing might feel absolutely necessary and even crucial in the moment, but are things ever perfectly dialed? We all tend to err on the side of doing more due to the fear of missing out or falling behind, then we are caught off guard when we're left injured, ill, or just plain burned out—and unable to enjoy or reap the rewards of all our hard work.

Also, it's usually when we most feel like we don't have time to rest or recover that we need it the most. Don't wait, embrace the time you do have to rest and recover.

Get out of your own way—rest now.

 ## Anchor Your Wins

If you're hung up on what's left to complete, reflect for a moment on what you've already accomplished. Acknowledge that it doesn't all have to happen at once, and that you don't need to get it all done in order to rest.

My Wins:

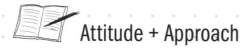

Attitude + Approach

Consider your relationship to recovery.

What does recovery mean to you?

When does it happen?

What does it look like?

What does it feel like?

Recovery is...

Rest, recovery, rejuvenation, reset, recharge... I use these terms interchangeably and, still, rest is so much more. What would you add to this list?

inward movement
gentle calming
processing
healing
repairing
absorption
compassionate being
settling

broadening perspective
a reset button
spacious boost
fuel

fresh eyes
relief
uplift
readiness

 ease

Doing

I'm guessing you might be here because you're fatigued? Well done for noticing. You've come to the right place.

Maybe you picked up this book because you're tired and wired, lying awake at night despite deep fatigue; you've hit a plateau in your marathon training and have lost the spring in your stride; that tightness in your calf has just become full-on Achilles tendonitis; or the strain of long desk hours is making your neck and back shout, "Code red!" Maybe it's become hard to ignore the steady upwelling of unease you feel?

Chances are, there's a lot of doing—going, making, working, caring—wrapped around your tiredness, or tension, or whatever words best describe your fatigue. Doing more, all the time, is a go-to distraction, a shadow comfort that disconnects you from yourself, inhibiting your ability to clearly recognize how you feel and what you need and, ultimately, to respond with rest in a meaningful way.

 Have you been turning away from yourself by ignoring your fatigue?

Doing Disguised as Recovery

It's ironic that recovery is often approached as another means of increasing output, a way to stay on the conveyor belt of busyness. How many people do you know who push it to the limit at work, and then jam-pack their "free time" with more? You know, the busy executive training for an Ironman, the fatigued athlete who goes to hot power yoga on their recovery day, the exhausted postpartum mother squeezing in fitness classes?

Or you might also fall into the doing trap. You've got to fit in that social event or get the workout done… despite being up most of the night with a toddler, or having to stay late at the office, or regardless of your knee pain. Or maybe you don't really have to do anything at all for at least a few minutes, and yet the inertia of doing keeps you finding ways to busy yourself. We give lip service to rejuvenation, but what we're really doing is finding more ways to push ourselves to be productive because we live in a culture that rewards doing.

We're so accustomed to doing that our endless action eclipses how we're feeling and what we really need. Moving in the opposite direction and allowing ourselves to *be* is completely outside our frame of reference. This mentality is a powerful force, leaving us overscheduled, overworked, and overstimulated… over the top and over the limit. Are you over it yet?

These are classic examples of the ways in which we extend ourselves fully and then look for recovery somewhere in between going for it and resting, rather than actually allowing ourselves to be at rest. This also demonstrates an increasingly prevalent ambivalence toward recovery and a fear of idleness.

The next time someone asks you what you did over the weekend, try casually sharing that you rested. That's it. *I just rested.* And then check out the reaction—a clear expression of surprise, confusion, even discomfort, settling onto the face of your exhausted acquaintance. This says a lot about our collective mentality about rest and recovery. Taking a break—and I don't mean a fancy spa trip or a weekend away— just because we're tired or, better yet, because we're being proactive about sustaining our energy, goes against the norm.

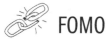 # FOMO

If you find yourself struggling to close your laptop at a reasonable hour, unwilling to reschedule your workout, or hesitant to take a rest day because you're afraid of missing out, losing momentum, or falling behind, consider the potential impact of pushing through at a time when you urgently need to rest. Needless to say, there's no medal for illness, injury, or burnout, and you're no use to anyone (especially not yourself) if you've overdone things.

FOMO, the fear of missing out, is real, especially when it feels like everyone around you is getting so much done and sprinting so hard. It's natural to feel like you're somehow not making the most of things when you pause. But by prioritizing the recovery you need, the only thing you'll miss out on is deep fatigue. Instead, consider the possibility of JOMO, the joy of missing out. You can confidently say no thank you to doing more, and be content in knowing how rewarding it is to honor what balance looks like for you.

It might also help to remind yourself that recovery is not an either/or situation. It's not like you have to sprint toward your goal to make meaningful progress. Rest doesn't take away from the main event, which could be running, cycling, writing a book, meeting big deadlines, or any other activities that you prioritize in your active lifestyle. However, rest is key to your success in the main event. So there's really nothing to miss out on by valuing your recovery time.

Sometimes we need to slow down in what feels like a radical way to keep moving forward.

 Do you really need to grit your teeth and power through? Or can you take a deeper breath and slow down?

Slow down significantly
to accelerate radically.

But My Workout Is Rejuvenating, You Say?

Yes, I hear you! Many people exercise to relieve stress, which is a healthy outlet. Indeed, active rest can be restorative. Physical activity helps you to get out of your head; it shifts your focus away from perceived stressors by pulling your attention into your body. It can literally help you to shake off stress, lingering tension, and pent-up emotion. While your workout usually feels refreshing, don't make the mistake of using more and more exercise simply as a break, distraction, or even an escape from stress, and don't confuse the relief you feel from shifting gears as recovery.

Exercise is by definition an output. While a great run, flow yoga class, or other physical movement can feel meditative or rejuvenating in the moment, it's not the same as restorative practice, and you shouldn't expect an outcome of recovery. You might notice the opposite, that your body feels even more fatigued than it did before that additional effort, or the angry hamstring you managed to ignore while you were in motion is now crying out for help, or that you are rushing into your next activity feeling stressed by the revelation that you have indeed passed up a chance to chill out.

While escaping into your favorite exercise might feel good temporarily, be aware of the additional buildup of fatigue that is likely to accompany that effort. Repeating this behavior over time risks hindering fitness and performance—and can even run you right into injury.

 Do you use exercise to escape? How might those additional outputs compromise your balance and well-being?

Frazzled or Fit?

It's always timely to acknowledge that frazzled is not fit. We often wear our busyness and related tiredness like a badge of honor, talking about how manic and utterly exhausting it all is. While most things worth doing require significant effort, and your accomplishments should be acknowledged and celebrated, you might ask yourself whether you're simply glorifying your busyness to fit into a society that expects it. Are you complaining about your fatigue or are you proud of it?

The consequences of doing too much, especially over a prolonged period of time, are unsustainable and often just plain overwhelming. Maybe you're noticing this on a daily basis, or feeling the effects of months, even years, of overextending. The result of overdoing can manifest as a sharp crescendo of stress or a deep valley of fatigue, and while it might feel like it's hitting you all at once, chances are it's been creeping up slowly, for some time. And the longer you ignore it or procrastinate on recovery by keeping busy, the more intense the results are likely to be and the longer they will take to remedy.

Most of us find ourselves in a convergence of at least a few of the scenarios I've mentioned. We live in a world that encourages us to do too much at all costs and leaves little to no time to make sense of it—no opportunity to reflect on or integrate what has happened. Our experiences are shaped by our excessive doing because this is where we point our attention, thoughts, and behavior, day in and day out.

When you force through fatigue, your mind and body will compensate for this imbalance in all kinds of less-than-ideal ways to keep you going and will continue to do so until all of the doing comes to a full stop. Doing becomes a coping mechanism, and while it might be useful when a deadline is looming, it's not sustainable.

As you endeavor to get it all done in all the different roles you play, stress and tension continue to build up in your mind and body, and the imbalance that accompanies relentless doing will eventually show up as illness, injury, and burnout. Endless doing creates real and often long-term consequences for health and well-being.

 Do you feel frazzled or fit? In what direction is all this doing fueling you?

A Break from Doing

Throughout each day are many moments when you can choose to do more, or pause and choose to take a break, or even to do a little bit less. When you fully inhabit a zone of doing, it takes awareness to practice moving in the other direction.

- The next time you find yourself organizing your time or schedule, pause.
- Take a deep breath.
- Notice the natural inclination to fill your time with doing—maybe an appointment is canceled at the last minute and you quickly find something else to slot into that time? Or you jump at the chance to squeeze in an extra errand?
- Take another deep breath and acknowledge that there's another zone, a movement away from doing.
- Choose to pause and be still when you can rather than initiating more action.

 Feel the difference after you've had a brief pause, as you move back into the flow of your day.

Create Space for Recovery

Consider the possibility of a more spacious schedule, which is more conducive to consistent, effective recovery. If this suggestion feels uncomfortable or overwhelming, it's probably a sign you're doing too much and will benefit immensely from prioritizing more space between your daily happenings.

You are responsible for creating space for yourself and modeling that for your colleagues, teammates, and family. No one can do it for you.

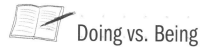

Doing vs. Being

Take a moment to consider how much you're actually doing—it's probably more than you realize.

Divide this circle into your doing and being, working and resting. What's on your very full plate? If you like, add some notes about what your main doing/being activities include.

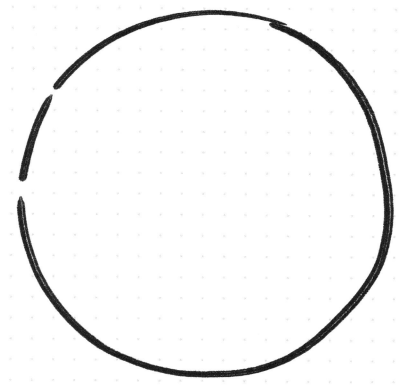

What kind of balance (or lack thereof) do you see?

How might that contribute to your fatigue?

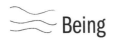 # Being

A path of less resistance starts with being. When we rest, we balance our doing with being, and this supports our longevity in all endeavors.

How do you undo the imbalance of overdoing it? And how much rest and recovery do you actually need? This is a question of balance. And, just as there isn't a tidy truth for achieving balance, your restorative needs will vary day to day.

There are many internal props, or coping mechanisms—adrenaline, structural compensation patterns, etc.—that hold us up and keep us going when we face mental and physical imbalance such as fatigue. When we are being, on purpose, we signal to these props that they can loosen their grip, helping to move us toward equilibrium. Being dismantles the rigid scaffolding of doing we so often build around ourselves so that we can settle into the balance that we are designed for. We'd be wise to practice this preemptively, rather than waiting for our intrinsic and often subconscious efforts to keep going to fail us and force a hard stop.

You're aware that recovery is important—rest is trending and the wellness marketplace is booming with everything from assisted stretching to float tanks to dedicated recovery centers, all promising to repair your overworked systems. And yet, most of us are still falling short in the rest space, and the irony of how much help we need to pause, rest, and just be—and not just for the sake of gain—shouldn't be lost.

Do you consider recovery to be as important as everything else that you do? Even so, when's the last time you approached rest with the same commitment as work?

Recovery is a crucial component of being a balanced and resilient human. And while the outcome of feeling and performing better is motivating, we need to unwire a few notions:

- We should rest for the sake of productivity or progression.
- We're somehow only worthy if we're always doing.
- We need permission to rest.

Developing a restorative mindset requires that you abandon these ways of thinking and unravel the notion that you must constantly produce. You need recovery not to achieve or to improve yourself, but rather to balance work and rest and to feel better. Decreasing doing requires some undoing—it requires you to be.

Permission granted—rest.

The Discomfort of Being

We get addicted to action in ways that can be counterproductive, especially in the long run. Whether your vice is saying yes to all invitations, lifting weights, or ticking things off your to-do list, the inertia of doing and its accompanying stimulation might feel like a high. Being amped up feels normal—but it's not. So it's no surprise if we feel some turbulence when presented with the opportunity to wind down. Being wound up is a familiar, even comfortable, zone, but is it good?

Busy for the sake of busy is not, in fact, a good thing, and further feeds into the collective mindset that it's not okay to stop and rest. It also employs a bit of forced positive thinking—*I'm okay! I can keep going!*—which further disconnects us from how we're really feeling and hinders our ability to respond and support ourselves in a timely manner. What's more timely is to normalize being.

 We're conditioned to do a lot and stay busy, but why? And to whose benefit?

Choose Balance

If any of this is making you feel uncomfortable, consider it affirmation that you need more rest. Finding the right balance between working and resting, doing and being, is ultimately your responsibility. You choose! Check your rest ambivalence. If you find any of these notions triggering, that might be indicative of your relationship with rest. Maybe, for example, you feel anxious that you're being idle or lazy when you take some time off. Or maybe you haven't even considered that space can be occupied by rest. Consider any emerging discomfort about the possibility of moving toward rest a nudge to explore a different, more balanced approach. Integrating more rest will likely feel better and be more sustainable when you give it a chance, and that is galvanizing.

It's okay to lighten your load.

 ## Be Brave

A certain amount of courage is required to do anything outside our comfort zones or usual frames of reference. We run at all kinds of challenges in life, and rest is no different. Going against your (and society's) habitual doing might feel disorienting, unfamiliar, or even scary—but that's okay. Don't shy away from the challenge. What matters is that you're brave in prioritizing and using your rest in the same way that you bravely commit to other pursuits. There is strength in taking a more balanced approach.

Rest is radical.

 Be Receptive to Rest

Accessing recovery is really difficult if you're not receptive to it. You've picked up this book, which signals some acknowledgment of rest's importance and your readiness to embrace recovery. Resistance and acceptance can coexist, side by side, and recognizing this is a useful shift in mindset, a win in itself. Now can you meet any resistance you have to resting with acceptance?

- Sit comfortably.
- Take a deep breath in… a slow breath out…
- Continue to deepen your breathing.
- Scan your body and notice any resistance to relaxation—this could be a tense muscle, a persistent thought, a feeling of agitation…
- Visualize those observations in whatever way they feel—a tight fist ready to fight back or a diver paralyzed in fear, unable to leap off the diving board. Conjure up a specific visual that illustrates the resistance you feel.

- Now move that visual in the opposite direction—see your palm opening or watch yourself bravely leaping into your recovery, by choice, free from anything holding you back.
- Continue to identify any lingering resistance, being as specific as possible, and see the alternative, embracing the possibility of unwinding that resistance.

Listen to your body.

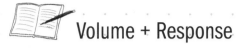
Volume + Response

Reflect on your current volume of activity and your resulting fatigue.

Why are you doing so much and keeping so busy?

Is your volume moving you forward? Or making you feel good?

Name a time when you were really fatigued and pushed through your planned activities anyway.

What did that feel like?

What was the outcome?

Name a time when you felt fully rested, effectively recovered.

What did that feel like?   *What was the outcome?*

You can do everything right (perfectionists, this is for you)—curate the best schedule, follow the perfect training plan, and eat all the right foods. But without fully embracing your mind and body's innate need for rest, and dedicating ample attention to it, you will miss out. The real value of rest is in actively absorbing all your hard work, coming into balance, and refueling to keep going.

If you don't value recovery and cultivate a restorative mindset, you lose.

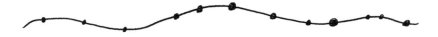

How do I know when to stop and rest?

Habit vs. Choice

Every day we are either consciously or unconsciously shaping our experience. It's worth considering whether your recovery or lack thereof is an unconscious habit or an intentional choice. Inertia is a powerful force, and our daily doing, making, and going leave little time for pausing, reflecting, and being. As we push through everything that needs to be done, it's easy to lose touch with how we feel in body and mind. Over time, this approach becomes habitual.

We also fail to decelerate because we're so caught up in keeping up that it becomes difficult to discern how much we're actually doing and how tired we really are (recall your notes from Doing vs. Being, page 37). Being amped up, experiencing a steady undercurrent of stress, feeling generally frazzled… we default to these ways of operating rather than naturally ebbing and flowing from work to rest—extending fully and relaxing completely—which is what we are designed to do.

Extend fully, relax completely—
don't get stuck in the middle.

To disrupt the momentum of your doing, you have to interrupt your regular pattern with rest and recovery—on purpose. Making this choice takes practice. Every time you choose rest when needed, you strengthen your ability to come into a more balanced state of being.

Disrupt Your Pattern

Become aware of your internal dialogue related to rest. Your approach is likely a pattern: you either notice and readily respond to fatigue, or you ignore it despite the consequences.

Use this quick practice to help unwire conditioning and more clearly discern how you want to respond to fatigue in the moment.

- Acknowledge when you feel the onset of tiredness, fatigue, sleepiness... or whatever best describes your need to rest.
- Notice any resistance you feel to acknowledging or responding to fatigue.
- Pause.
- Place one hand on your heart or anywhere on your body that feels intuitive or comforting.
- Close your eyes and take a deep breath.
- Say to yourself, gently, "stop."
- Stay here for a moment, breathing deeply, acknowledging how you're feeling—and, in doing so, momentarily calming your systems.

Repeat whenever fatigue pops up, acknowledging and softening your reaction to your need for respite.

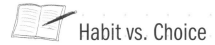

Habit vs. Choice

Think about whether your recovery or lack thereof is driven by habit or choice.

How do you respond to your mind and body's need for rest?

Are you avoiding or resisting recovery?

Why might that be?

Is this an unconscious habit or an intentional choice?

How does it feel to practice being more receptive to rest, and to take a more restorative approach to addressing fatigue?

Notice

Pay attention and, with practice, you will notice when it's time to rest and recover. This attunement is the gateway to rejuvenation and is critical for protecting your mental health, preventing injuries, and finding balance.

Your mind and body's requests for respite can sneak up in subtle yet distinct ways. Maybe you need 20 minutes to compose an email that would usually take 2 minutes, or your legs feel like lead when you're walking up the stairs. So many chronic issues originate in seemingly small ways—an upwelling of tiredness, the strange sensation in your ankle, that tension in your upper back… without noticing those signs, how can you possibly address them?

The simple gesture of noticing can be deeply restorative in itself, a gentle act of meeting yourself in the moment, coming into the present, allowing yourself to be here, now… While this book offers a variety of tools to support your restorative practice, keep in mind that pausing—anytime, anywhere—to check in with yourself and to notice how you are is one of the most important and available self-supporting practices.

Before we consider what to do (coming up in the next chapter), we first have to know when to stop doing and start being, and we find that discernment by noticing how we are in body and mind, day to day and moment to moment.

Attention holds the power to move us toward balance.

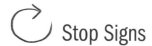

Stop Signs

Here are some common signs that your mind and body will give you when it's time to stop and rest:

- Your breathing is erratic.
- You're mentally foggy, unfocused, or feeling out of control.
- You have a hard time regulating your emotions.
- Your patience and tolerance for coworkers, family, and everyday obstacles are waning.
- Your usually efficient or automatic tasks are taking longer and becoming frustrating.
- You find it difficult to maintain a broad perspective.
- Your workouts are adding to your everyday stress rather than helping you to manage it.
- You're going through the motions and not really getting any benefit from your training.
- You feel like you've hit a performance plateau.
- You find it difficult to wind down even when the opportunity for rest presents itself.
- You feel exhausted yet have trouble sleeping.

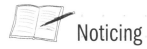 Noticing

Notice how you are and what you need.

What do you notice in your mind and body? What thoughts and sensations are coming up?

Were you aware of these things before slowing down and paying attention?

Rest Recap

Hopefully, by now you're starting to feel more open to the power of rest and recovery. You know that it's important, it's active, and it's readily available to you; and you're recognizing when to pivot into rejuvenation. You're ready to activate rest in your everyday life.

- Rest and recovery is a practice.
- Recovery is for all of us—you hold the power to create accessible entry points for yourself.
- You have time to rest.
- Doing should be matched with being—it's a balance.
- You're not missing out on anything by claiming the rest that you need.
- Rest requires receptivity.
- You choose—make intentional restorative choices or fall victim to the habit of underrecovering.
- Your body will tell you everything you need to know about what it needs. Pay attention—notice.

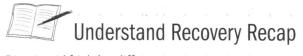

Understand Recovery Recap

Pause and feel the difference.

What's changed for you—even if it's subtle—since you first opened this book?

How are rest and recovery landing with you at this point in your journey?

What do you find the most motivating and/or inspiring about real recovery?

Now that you've explored the key elements of cultivating a restorative mindset, how would you answer these questions in the context of your own life?

Why should I rest and recover?

How do I know when to stop and rest?

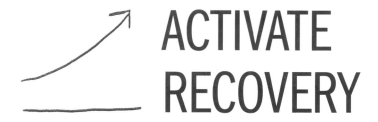

ACTIVATE RECOVERY

Learn to Use Rest

As you continue to develop your restorative mindset, you'll fine-tune your ability to recognize when it's time to stop working and to start resting (see Stop Signs, page 52). But once you stop, what should you do? This is when it's time to activate real recovery with contextual practice in order to connect the dots of how to make rest work for you.

Remember—recovery is not automatic. The concept of activating rest might seem counterintuitive. Just because you've stopped work doesn't mean you're not working. Don't be surprised if you find yourself at a loose end, uncomfortable, or unsettled when you close your laptop or pull off your sneakers and don't feel immediate relief. It can take time to unwind. We're so stimulated and engaged that when left to "just rest," we commonly feel a bit stuck—tense, tight, stiff—somewhere in between working and resting, rather than smoothly settling into the recovery that we need. You won't find real rejuvenation in the middle.

Meaningful recovery is a matter of balance, and while there's a natural tension between going and stopping, we have to cultivate the skill that enables us to fully release ourselves to rest in the same way that we fully extend ourselves to work. That's where recovery activation comes in.

 ## I'm Not Good at It

The key mental and physical recovery tools I offer in this book are based on meditation and restorative yoga. People tell me all the time that they don't meditate because they can't quiet their mind, or they're not good at yoga because they're too inflexible. In either case, I usually respond by asking how often they practice. The usual response: avoidance. Things that are unfamiliar, or outside your usual frame of reference based on your habitual use or activity, are bound to feel uncomfortable or even like you're not doing them right. That's okay.

There's a certain comfort that accompanies the familiar discomfort of pushing yourself to your limits. Modern life demands a high volume, and you're accustomed to responding to that. The confusion and related discomfort of doing something beyond your usual mode of operation, well, that's something entirely different.

Recovery might not feel good at first. Let's just accept that up front. That being said, it's not about good and bad. It's about balance and locating equanimity with whatever comes up for you. You might find that you need to increase your tolerance for resting. You wouldn't expect running three miles to feel good if you haven't put on sneakers in a year, would you? So why would you expect intentional rest to feel natural, or even pleasant? Consider discomfort a sign that you're in the right zone, one that will force you to grow in a healthy way.

It's a little bit like when you're training a muscle and it starts to shake or tremble. That awkward trembling is actually your brain's confusion caused by a discrepancy between what it thinks is possible and what is actually possible, based on your habitual use of that muscle. With time and attention, you can close this gap between perception and reality.

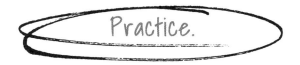

Practice.

Move into Relaxation

What is the difference between "being on" and "switching off"? How can you more effectively engage fully and then relax completely, and in doing so sustain a balance that supports your well-being? Begin in familiar territory—your body. It can be helpful to go to both extremes to become aware of the ways in which we often get caught in the middle, neither fully engaged or relaxed. You can't move into recovery if you only go halfway. Use this quick practice to feel the difference.

- Make tight fists, squeezing as hard as you can.
- Now relax completely, allowing your palms to gently open.
- Pause and feel the difference.

Try the same thing in other areas of your body:

- Your jaw: Clench your teeth and then soften.
- Your belly: Hollow your center tightly and then release.
- Your glutes: Squeeze your butt firmly and then let it go.
- Your whole body: Tense and tighten from head to toe and then let it all go.

When you practice in this way, you might discover that some areas are more difficult to release than others, which is common for most of us. This noticing gives you a lot of information about where you're likely holding tension. For example, maybe it's easy to relax your butt muscles, but you can't seem to loosen your tight jaw. As you gain this awareness, you'll know which areas are your own practice must-haves.

Extend fully, relax completely—
don't get stuck in the middle.

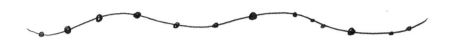

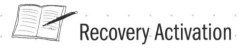

Recovery Activation

Practice recognizing the difference between engaging and relaxing, and try extending fully in both directions. Use this awareness to start unwinding habitual tension.

What areas of your body do you find difficult to relax?

Where do you notice yourself holding tension even as you try to unwind?

Why might that be? Can you allow those places to soften and move toward rest?

When I stop, what should I do?

Even as rest is gaining attention, so many of the practices offered are output-focused and relate to the physical body and outer appearance—everything from hot power yoga that "burns off excess" to compression boots that ease muscle swelling. It's somewhat ironic that so many restorative activities first focus on muscles, even though muscles naturally recover quicker because they receive direct blood flow. While many of these modalities can be useful in aiding the recovery process, they employ an outside-in focus and easily distract and further disconnect us from how we're really feeling inside.

There's a deeper level of life load–induced fatigue that you can't foam roll your way out of, and by fixating on your physical body and external factors, you'll be prone to further overdoing it. Instead, consider resourcing one of the most readily available internal tools you possess to facilitate your own healing and support your resilience—your nervous system.

Remember, this is less about self-improvement and more about meeting yourself where you are.

Balance Your Nervous System

Your nervous system includes your central nervous system, comprising your brain and spinal cord, and your peripheral nervous system, featuring nerves that extend throughout your body. While, functionally speaking, you're probably most familiar with your somatic nervous system, which feels sensation and signals your body to move through space, there's another part called the autonomic nervous system. This comprises your sympathetic and parasympathetic nervous systems. It regulates your body's instinctive, unconscious actions, influences the function of your internal organs, and regulates many bodily functions, such as heart rate, digestion, blood pressure, and respiration—all of which keep you going and moving forward and play a crucial role in movement, exertion, and ultimately performance.

Generally speaking, your nervous system facilitates communication between your brain and internal organs, creating a dialogue between your mind and your musculoskeletal system. While you might assume your brain is the boss at all times, it's actually a two-way street, as your body equally informs your mind, harmonized in an ongoing feedback loop. This is why it's so crucial (and an accurate instruction) to *listen to your body*.

To regulate effectively, your nervous system asks that you be ready to get up and go, while equally capable of settling down at any given moment (see Move into Relaxation, page 60). Admittedly, this can be really hard when you're constantly running on the treadmill of life. Becoming aware of these polarities and opening yourself to the ongoing conversation that's happening between your brain and body are good places to start.

Pause and Feel the Difference

Inertia is a powerful force. Often we do things at such high volume and speed that we lose track of how our actions affect us and how we're really feeling. The same goes for restorative practice. If you rush or go through the motions without really paying attention to what you're doing, you won't get the full benefit.

When you *slow down, breathe deeply, and pay attention*, you become more aware of the effects of your practice. What you've done has a chance to land. This is a practice in itself and a motivating force that will help you to stay with it. Between stretches or sides of the body, and as you end a practice, pause long enough to notice the impact of what you've done, not just in your muscles or thoughts, but in your overall state—this is your nervous system talking to you. Then, perhaps any positive shifts feel more available to you, and you can use them to set the tone going forward.

 How might your practice set the tone or shape your intention as you move forward?

Use this feeling to set the tone.

GO! vs. Stop

Your nervous system sounds the alarm by way of a chemical stress response, often referred to as fight-or-flight, when you're confronted with stressful situations. Your sympathetic nervous system (SNS) triggers a reaction in which blood pressure increases to supply more oxygen to your brain and muscles and all your systems are optimized for you to defend yourself or run for your life. Your focus narrows to meet the challenge. This is incredibly useful if you're attacked in a dark alley (hopefully, an unlikely happening). Or running from a pack of stray dogs (even less likely). Or, more likely, when you're rushing to meet that end-of-day deadline or kicking hard for a new personal best in the last 400 meters of your race.

On the opposite end of the spectrum, your relaxation response is governed by your parasympathetic nervous system (PNS)—this allows you to rest and digest, to settle down and absorb what has happened. Since your nervous system is designed for self-preservation, your PNS should kick in once stressful events have passed, slowing your heart rate, aiding digestion, and returning you to a baseline of calm. It broadens your perspective and helps you to be more aware of where you are so that you can more clearly discern the most appropriate course of action, rather than just react. Activating your PNS increases your resilience and helps you to more easefully manage whatever comes at you.

Sympathetic nervous system (SNS): *GO!*
Parasympathetic nervous system (PNS): *Stop.*

The problem is that because we are doing so much, all the time, and at such speed, we get stuck in fight-or-flight mode and struggle to wind down. As a result, the SNS response is more easily triggered by normal day-to-day happenings, like the chaos of the morning school run, hurrying to get a workout in, or triaging a full email inbox or a device full of notifications.

When you're in this frame of mind, your brain might perceive failing to meet your deadline or desired pace the same way it perceives an actual threat like getting mugged. Being late for your meeting because you're stuck in traffic suddenly feels like a matter of life or death. While it can be useful to get fired up to rise to meet challenges and get a certain amount of things done, getting amped up in gridlock confuses your body with unnecessary stress and deprives you of the opportunity to spend that time in a more relaxed state. The physiological design of the nervous system is disrupted by the pace of life. Stress management might be a big motivator of your active lifestyle, but without consistent, effective PNS activation, you're merely creating a vicious cycle of SNS stimulation.

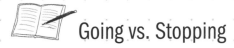 ## Going vs. Stopping

Consider your time typically spent going (SNS), compared to stopping (PNS).

Divide this circle into your working versus relaxing, comparing when you're stimulated to when you're at rest. Make notes about any particular activities that relate to each.

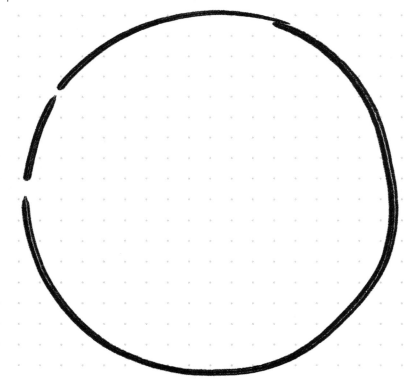

What do you see?

What does your go vs. stop balance look like?

An Inside-Out Approach

Soothing your nervous system promotes recovery. It helps you transition from a heightened, often overstimulated state to a healing state that's more conducive to rejuvenation and sustainable well-being. Because your nervous system is so intimately involved with your ability to recover efficiently and effectively, what's missing is an inside-out approach.

It's less thinking and more noticing, and it asks you to engage your felt sense, also known as "interoception." This is your internal sense that answers questions like, *How am I?* and *How do I feel?* It helps you to discern when you are feeling hungry or hot or, most crucially, when you are tired. This noticing supports healthy nervous system regulation, and maintaining this awareness facilitates an ever-important and ongoing processing of sensations and actions as you move through your days.

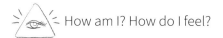 How am I? How do I feel?

Less thinking, more noticing.

Interoception is a particularly important aspect of recovery, because prompting your awareness of how you are sparks your growing understanding of when it's time to stop. The more you use interoception, the easier it becomes to discern how you're doing and to respond with rest in the moments when you need it most.

Even knowing this, accessing felt sense might seem elusive, which is likely because it's outside our usual frame of reference. So what should you do? *Slow down, breathe deeply, pay attention. Notice.* (More noticing practices coming up in Mental Focus, page 73.) Give yourself a handhold by creating clear entry points that calm and center you, rather than leaving yourself to flop and fidget when you try to unwind. While this is an incredibly unique and personal journey, there are some tried-and-true tools to create the entry points needed to support meaningful recovery.

Let's create some doorways. Try them out and see what feels best to move through.

Notice.

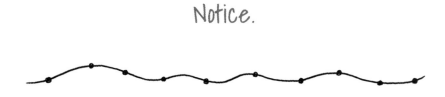

Notice

Take a moment now to engage your interoception, your felt-sense ability to recognize how you are. You'll probably find that you need to slow down to do this, which is totally expected. Consider slowing down a good thing—it allows you to notice.

- Sit comfortably.
- Take a deep breath in… a slow breath out…
- Continue to deepen your breathing.
- Slowly scan your body, starting with your toes and moving all the way to your head…
- What do you notice? What do you feel?
- Sensations, overall mood and energy, thoughts… take your time and be specific, letting go of any reaction to judge or turn away from what comes up.
- Stay with it until you're more clear about how you are and how you feel.

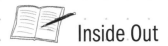 Inside Out

When you slow down and pay attention, interoception is easier to engage. If you don't often pose these questions to yourself, don't be surprised if the answers are unclear. That's okay, and a sign it might be time to ask more often.

What do you notice when you engage your felt-sense?

How are you?

How do you feel right now?

Your Tools

It's time to develop and activate your restorative skill set. You're ready to rest! It's easy to schedule recovery; what's more difficult is to activate it in a meaningful way. Thankfully, you have practical tools at the ready to serve your restorative processes. For the sake of practicality, we'll use your two most readily available resources as entry points; they happen to be the same systems we're here to reset—your mind and your body. Mental and physical rest and recovery go hand in hand.

Mental Focus

Meditation is mental focus training that supports us to relax and recharge so that we can feel and perform our best. To meditate is to focus your mind on something—it creates a way into your attention, and helps you to settle into the present moment, which is one of the most crucial aspects of restorative practice. The benefits of meditation are expansive: it's a practice that improves focus and attentional capacity, increases emotional stability and regulation, strengthens immunity, improves sleep, and so much more. It's a powerful practice of being.

Whereas we tend to focus on the physical body when it comes to recovery, mental rest is just as important as physical. You can use all the stretches, ice, and massages, but if your head isn't in the game—you're still busy planning, solving, and fixing—your capacity to recharge will remain limited.

By settling your attention inward, you can more clearly notice the all-important signals your mind, body, and nervous system constantly give you about what's needed to support yourself to be well in any given moment. This noticing is crucial for tending to yourself in a sustainable way.

Meditation is...

It's no surprise that mental focus isn't easy given that our attention is so often scattered and difficult to control, like marbles on a plate. This is why we meditate—to gather our attention, resettling ourselves into ourselves, in the present, which is a more easeful state of being. Despite any stereotypes the term conjures or notions you might have based on previous negative experiences, there is no "good" or "bad" meditation, it's really just about showing up and staying with your practice rather than how it might look or unfold.

Now let's set aside the word "meditation" because it can be a bit intimidating. People say all the time that they can't meditate because they can't quiet their mind. And I find so often that the problem isn't that they can't, but rather they haven't given themselves the opportunity to experience it. They haven't stayed with it long enough to see what's beneath any initial confusion or discomfort that naturally accompanies doing something new or different (see I'm Not Good at It, page 58). Time and reps are needed to activate and strengthen the skill, as they are for most things.

"It's not what you might think it is," I usually respond. For example, I meditate most days, and a typical morning practice often looks something like this for me, as I'm seated on a sofa cushion on my living room floor surrounded by Legos:

Do I hear my son coughing?
I wonder what the weather's doing today…

Take a deep breath in…
a slow breath out…
Continue to deepen your breathing.

Coconut porridge sounds nice for breakfast, hmmm, or are we out of coconut?
Inhale deeply…

Why is my jaw so tight?
Exhale completely…

My son's homework is due today… or is it my daughter's that needs handing in?
A deep breath in…
a slow breath out…

That feeling of being perfectly windswept and sandy after a day at the beach…
Maybe if I move that 1 p.m. meeting, I'll have enough time to get that piece of writing done.
Just inhale…
Just exhale…

This carries on for what feels like an eternity. Thoughts rise and recede, a seemingly endless flow of memories, concerns, and plans.

Without slowing my breathing, it all seems to blur together, a dizzying swirl of past and future, the soup of an ever-busy mind. I've learned that it settles if I simply notice rather than attach or create stories around the details that arise, if I patiently stay with it, with myself.

It turns out meditating isn't about silencing yourself—it's about staying with yourself. This is the practice. Don't worry about whether it's "good" or "working," just show up and stay with it.

 ## Activate Mental Focus

Meditation is a practice of noticing what comes up for you and gently refocusing your mind into the present moment.

- Sit comfortably.
- Take a deep breath in… a slow breath out…
- Continue to deepen your breathing.
- Notice what's on your mind, any questions, cares, or concerns…
- Without judging or trying to solve or fix, acknowledge each thought and come back to the present moment where you are simply sitting and breathing, being here— no good or bad, everything just as it is.

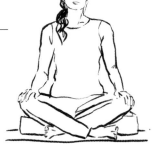

- Continue noticing then gently guiding yourself back into the moment.

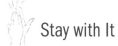 ## Stay with It

You've probably noticed by now that it's hard to think about nothing. It can be surprisingly uncomfortable or even agitating to be still and mentally quiet. A parade of thoughts is likely to surface, a deep restlessness or unexpected emotion. That's okay. Practice letting things be as they are, moment by moment.

Stay with yourself.

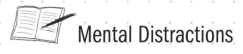

Mental Distractions

Distractions are normal and to be expected. Think about what kind of things come up for you when you create space to settle your mind.

Where's your head at when it's recovery time?

Where does your mind tend to wander, and what impact does that have on your rest?

What distractions or challenges have you noticed if or when you've tried any kind of meditation?

Meditative Tools

A number of powerful sensory tools are available to focus the mind and ease the mental chaos that so often inhibits our ability to calm down and rest. These tools include breath, mantra, visualization, and felt sense—all clear entry points to your attention and to noticing. Use each of these highly accessible tools like a GPS to soothe your nervous system, thereby connecting your brain and body to active recovery.

One tool or approach might feel easier than others, more helpful for connecting you to rest. Start there and continue to explore the other entry points, knowing that they, too, can bring you relief as you practice and learn to wield them.

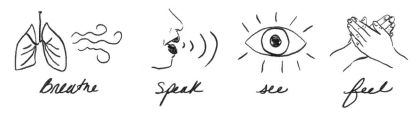

Breathe   Speak   see   feel

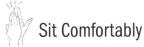 # Sit Comfortably

We're here to rest and recharge, not to further strain ourselves. Sitting shouldn't be rigid or feel hard, or affect your ability to focus—if you're dying for it to be over, chances are you haven't set yourself up well.

Despite the vast amount of time we spend sitting in chairs, on sofas, in cars, and more, our bodies aren't really designed to sit in this way. The one place we should be able to sit with relative ease is on the floor—think of how easily a child can sit on the floor, legs crossed, spine tall—but this posture has become less and less accessible to many of us due to muscular imbalances caused by prolonged chair sitting. Sore back, hunched shoulders, tight hips… have you noticed the effects?

When sitting for restorative practice (or any time), lengthening tall helps to neutralize the spine, which optimizes your posture and breathing. Your body supports your breath, and your breath supports your body. This can be difficult and uncomfortable if your spine is rounding forward and/or you're not supported from beneath.

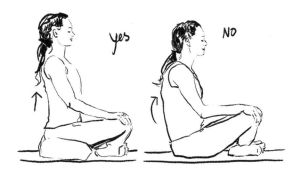

yes

NO

Try these options to find your most comfortable position, and remember that the more you sit, the more comfortable it will become, the more natural it will feel, and the more readily you will be able to relax into your practice:

- **On a prop:** Sit on a bolster, pillow, or folded blanket so that your hips are supported and you can lengthen your spine tall. Loosely cross your legs or extend them in front of you for knee comfort.

- **At the wall:** If sitting tall is difficult, take your prop (bolster, pillow, or blanket) to the wall for added support so you have support to lean into.

- **In a chair:** If hip or low back discomfort makes sitting on the floor unbearable, sit tall on the edge of a chair.

Stillness is a restorative practice.

↻ Extended Exhalation

Lengthening your exhale has a profound calming effect on your nervous system, helping you to slow your heart rate and relax.

- Sit comfortably.
- Take a deep breath in… a slow breath out…
- Continue to deepen your breathing.
- Inhale as you count 1-2-3-4.
- Exhale as you count 1-2-3-4-5-6.
- Breathe in for 4.
- And out for 6.
- Keep slowing it down, and see if you can lengthen your exhale to 8 counts or more.
- Continue for a few minutes, or until you feel more calm and settled.

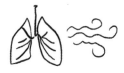

Just breathe in… Just breathe out…

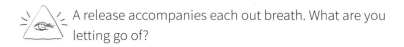 A release accompanies each out breath. What are you letting go of?

Activate recovery with your breath.

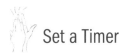 ## Set a Timer

I leave the duration of many practices in this book open-ended, with instruction such as "Continue for a few minutes, or until you feel more calm and settled." How long you practice is up to you and will naturally fluctuate based on how you're feeling and practicalities such as location or time available. That being said, setting a timer can be really helpful, freeing you from wondering what time it is or how long you've been at it. Just be sure to let go of any urge to clock watch.

Mantra Meditation

Your favorite mantra or positive affirmation provides a clear focal point for your attention, helping to anchor you in the present and bridge the gap between how you feel right now and how you want to feel (rested). Use a restorative mantra to help you wind down and relax anytime.

- Select your mantra, ideally one that is relevant for recovery, for example, *I can rest, I am calm* or *I am here now* or *Just this*.
- Sit comfortably.
- Take a deep breath in… a slow breath out…
- Continue to deepen your breathing.
- Inhaling, say in your head, *I can rest.*
- Exhaling, say, *I am calm.*
- Inhale: *I can rest.*
- Exhale: *I am calm.*
- Continue for a few minutes, or until you feel more calm and settled.

I am here now.

Restful Inventory Visualization

Take a brief inventory of your output and then visualize the balancing input that happens when you slow down, breathe deeply, pay attention... and rest.

- Sit comfortably.
- Take a deep breath in... a slow breath out...
- Continue to deepen your breathing.
- Take a few moments to review your agenda, tasks, and mental to-do lists... Where are you? What are you doing? Let your mind wander around your happenings...
- Pause and take a deep breath.
- Now take a few moments to visualize the restful pauses before, in between, and after all the key events of your day. Where are you? What are you doing? Locate the moments of respite available to you.
- Pause and feel the spaciousness that accompanies the possibility of resting throughout your day.

Set your sight on how you want to be-rested.

Feeling Meditation

Use the sensation of your breath as a feeling anchor. Bringing your focus to the distinct sensations of your breath entering and exiting your nose helps to add a more tangible, tactile quality to your breathing and ultimately to your mental focus.

- Sit comfortably.
- Take a deep breath in… a slow breath out…
- Continue to deepen your breathing.
- Become more aware of your breathing—its pattern, pace, and depth as it is now—just breathe.
- With your mouth gently closed, focus on your nostrils and notice the sensations of your breath entering and leaving your nose.
- Without trying to change anything, continue to feel your breath.
- If distraction arises, refocus on the tactile sensations of your breath moving through your nostrils with each inhale and exhale.
- Continue for a few moments, until you feel more attuned to the sensation of your breath.

Get out of your thinking mind
and into your feeling body.

Use Your Breath

In any given moment, the quality of your breath will tell you everything you need to know about your interior state. While shallow, erratic breathing (or even holding your breath) is indicative of stress, tension, or fatigue, deep steady breathing tends to accompany a more calm, relaxed state. Use your breath to connect to balance anytime, anywhere.

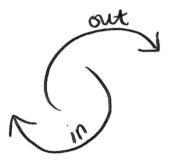

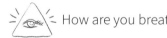 How are you breathing? Are you holding your breath?

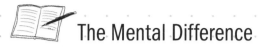 ## The Mental Difference

Take the time to feel the difference in your mind, whether obvious or subtle, after mental focus practices.

When you pause and feel the difference after your practice, what do you notice?

Can you feel any effects as you continue to move through your day?

Which of the meditative tools (breathe, speak, see, feel) do you connect with? What best supports your mind to settle and feel at rest?

Physical Relaxation

Modern life results in an array of physical imbalances, and recovery helps us to neutralize our biomechanics (the way all your parts, including your bones, connective tissue, and muscles, are engineered to work together). Restorative yoga is a physical relaxation practice that calms the body and mind. It's a restful approach to yoga that decreases tension, boosts breath capacity, increases circulation and blood flow to your internal organs, improves immune system function, and more. It encourages deep relaxation and promotes physical and mental recovery.

Bear in mind that when it comes to recovery, not all yoga is created equal. While all valuable in different ways, many styles of modern yoga are physically demanding and can be overly aggressive for a frazzled, overstimulated mind, and a fatigued, imbalanced body. While you might think that a power yoga class is the perfect way to wind down a frenetic week, ask yourself, *Is this just another means to push myself?* Remember that the last thing you need is another effort to power through (see Doing Disguised as Recovery, page 29). Instead, consider using yoga as a tool to retreat from mental and physical demands so that you can effectively recharge.

While traditional restorative yoga uses props such as blankets and cushions to support the body, in this book I offer solutions that require little to no propping to make the postures as practical and accessible as possible. Explore restorative yoga and additional propping as your time and interest allow.

Open Your Mat

An open yoga mat or cushion on the floor is a powerful visual cue to prompt a reset in a moment that you'd ordinarily pass right by. While props aren't required for restorative practice, you might find that having a mat open and ready—winking at you!—as you walk by is a reminder to use a favorite stretch or to pause and take a deep breath.

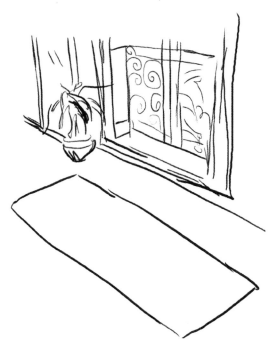

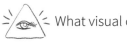 What visual cues prompt you to rest?

Activate Physical Relaxation

Although rest isn't easy, it doesn't have to be so hard. One of the simplest ways to activate physical rest is to lie down, allowing your body to stretch out and be supported by the ground beneath you. Have you considered the possibility of lying down not just at bedtime or when all the work is done, but anytime you're feeling tired? Better yet, how about a little lie-down as a proactive reboot whenever you find a pocket of time? Sounds a bit radical, doesn't it? It is, and that's why it works so well.

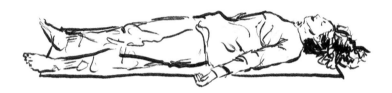

- Lie down on the floor on either a rug or a mat.
- Extend your legs long and rest your arms open, palms up.
- Notice the places where your body is in contact with the floor—heels, calves, glutes, back, shoulders, elbows, backs of the palms, back of the head…
- Let your bones drop and feel the support beneath you.
- Spend a few minutes here, continuing to let your body drop into the ground and rest.

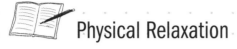

Physical Relaxation

Think about how you encourage and facilitate physical relaxation.

What physical activities support your body's rejuvenation?

When does your physical body feel the most rested and recharged?

In what activities, however well intended for recovery, do you find yourself having to push through?

Does pushing through "rest" make you feel recovered?

Physical Relaxation Tools

A few key approaches can help to encourage your body into a restful state and facilitate rejuvenation. Depending on how you're feeling and what you've been doing, consider inverting, grounding, or opening postures; or gentle mobilization can be appropriate. Use each of these practical tools to bring rest, ease, and balance to your body in the time you have on hand.

Different approaches will suit different contexts. It makes sense to stand up and have a little wiggle if you've been sitting at your desk for a few hours, whereas a legs-up-the-wall session is timely when you're at home winding down. Use these practices as different entry points to physical ease, and consider how and where they best fit into the practicalities of your day.

 ## Invert

Rest's classic call to action, to put your feet up, is always timely. When you sit, fluid and stagnation build up, especially in your lower body. Literally putting your body in the opposite direction—reaching your legs skyward and getting your lower extremities above your heart—helps to recirculate blood and any excess fluid in the legs, eases stagnation from sitting, and so much more. Get off your seat and feet, and move your legs up whenever you can.

↻ Legs Up the Wall

I call this setup "the boss" because when it comes to recovery, it is. So much active recovery in one simple posture! Legs up the wall recirculates the blood and excess fluid, opens the hamstrings, relaxes the low back and feet, and more.

- Lie on your back and extend your legs up the wall, moving as far back as needed so that your back feels comfortable.
- Bend your knees slightly and turn your feet away from each other.
- Rest your arms open, palms up.
- Breathe deeply and stay for 5–15 minutes.

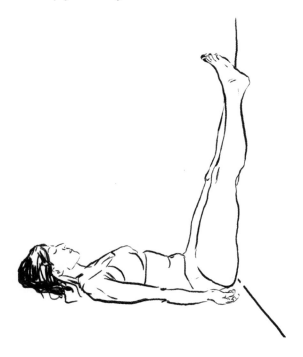

Add Additional Support

To boost your recovery, put a cushion or bolster under your butt and loop a strap or belt around your calves so that they are held in place. Use additional props as needed in any restorative posture to ensure you feel supported so that your body can be at rest.

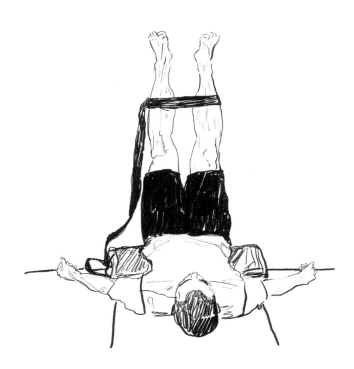

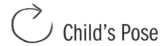 # Child's Pose

This restorative classic is like giving yourself a warm hug, and it eases shoulder, back, and hip stiffness. It's also an impactful calming gesture when you are feeling frazzled.

- Kneel with your legs hip-width apart, keeping your shins parallel.
- Lengthen your torso down onto your thighs.
- Reach your arms forward, palms down, or rest them back along your sides, palms up.
- Rest your forehead on the floor or on a yoga block or cushion.
- Stay for 10+ deep breaths.

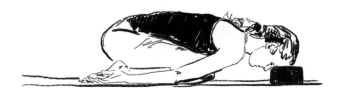

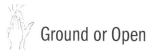 ## Ground or Open

There is a physical contraction that usually accompanies fatigue. Muscles tighten and shorten, causing postural imbalance. Accumulated strain and tension rounds our bodies forward. Picture it: you've been sitting at your desk for over three hours, your neck strained from reaching your head toward your computer screen, your shoulders and upper back rounded forward as you type…

It's in these cases that restorative postures ask us to move in the opposite direction—to open the body—in order to find ease and reset this growing imbalance so that physical contraction doesn't become habitual and cause long-term problems. Setups that lengthen and open the front of the body are most appropriate in countering physical contraction by helping to reestablish space in your body.

Alternatively, in situations where you are feeling frazzled, a calming and grounding gesture will serve you best. Forward bends, for example, are naturally introspective shapes and help us to move our attention inward and to settle down.

 When do you feel like you need to settle down and ground? When do you feel like you need to lift and open?

Open = Create Space

 ## Breathe over Bolster

Lying back over a prop lifts and opens the front of your body, which is so often shortened and tight from sitting. This also facilitates deeper breathing, a key to rest and recovery. This posture is super relaxing because you gain that opening without having to do any work, and your prop supports your overstretched back body to relax and settle back into a more neutral state.

- Sit down, pull a bolster or stacked cushions lengthwise against your butt.
- Extend your legs or bring the soles of your feet together, dropping your thighs apart.
- Lie back over the prop, keeping your butt on the floor.
- Rest your arms open, palms up.
- Breathe deeply and stay for 5 to 15 minutes.

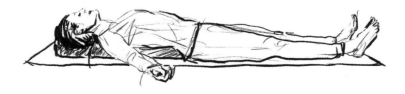

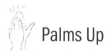 ## Palms Up

There is a natural tendency to turn our palms toward the floor when lying down, which mirrors the common postural imbalance of rounded forward shoulders due to tight chest muscles from sitting, training, child carrying, and more. The muscles internally rotate (turn in) the upper arm bones. If you're standing or sitting, for example, with your arms along your sides and you turn your palms to face back, you'll notice your posture hunch forward slightly.

Instead, externally rotate (turn out) your upper arm bones so your palms face up or forward, which opens the chest and helps the shoulder blades move back and down into their intended homes, supporting better posture and healthier biomechanics. Keep in mind that if your pecs are particularly tight, the backs of your palms might not easily touch the floor when you lie down. When left suspended with nothing to rest on, they place excess strain on your shoulders, so it's important that you find an arm placement that allows your knuckles to rest heavily on the floor.

Keep adjusting until you find a comfortable, palm-up position, and practice making this your default any time you lie down, which will ultimately help to balance your standing posture as well.

Hip Circles

Feeling stiff and lethargic? Sometimes gentle mobility is the best remedy for fatigue, especially after prolonged sitting. Wiggle all your parts and they'll work better. A simple movement addresses this reality and promotes better circulation and, with it, revitalized energy.

- Stand with your feet slightly wider than hip-width distance and your feet turned out a little.
- Put your hands on your hips and move your waist around in big circles, keeping your knees slightly bent.
- Notice how your hips and back feel, and then spread your awareness more broadly down toward your lower legs and feet, and up toward your shoulders and your neck, expanding your circles so that your whole body is participating in this gentle mobilization.
- Continue for 5 to 10 circles, and then switch directions.

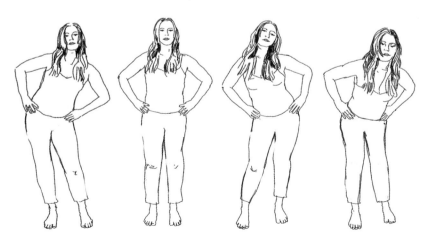

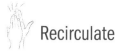 ## Recirculate

So much of what we perceive as more or better energy is, in fact, better circulation. Every human needs to recover from sitting and the body stiffness and imbalance, tension, and stagnation that result. Not all physical recovery has to be stretch-led.

Gentle movement also helps to increase fluidity, which is the ability to move with optimal power and minimal dysfunction, and equates to an energizing ease of movement. Mobilizing the body helps muscles, surrounding tissues, and joints to become more fluid. It also works to ease stiffness and restore range of motion, promoting full-body recovery and boosting energy.

In this case, rest is a literal movement and is particularly beneficial after prolonged sitting. While you might feel fatigued by desk strain and be longing for a nap, sometimes the most rejuvenating pause is to *gently* move your way into balance.

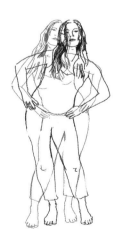

Better circulation = more energy

 How do you feel after you get up and move around, even if you don't really feel like doing so?

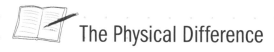

The Physical Difference

Take the time to feel the difference in your body, whether obvious or subtle, after physical relaxation practice.

When you pause and feel the difference after your practice, what do you notice?

Can you feel any effects as you continue to move through your day?

Which approach to physical relaxation (invert, ground, open, mobilize) best supports your body to feel settled and at rest?

Rest Recap

You're activating rest—yes! At this point, you know why it's important to stop and rest, and how to know when it's time. Now you're building your understanding of what to do. Keep using the practices in this chapter to fine-tune your awareness, soothe your nervous system, and move your mind and body into more effective rest.

- Recovery might not feel "good" at first—accept that this is okay!
- Balancing your nervous system is a crucial aspect of recovery.
- While our systems are designed to engage fully and relax completely, too often we try to find rest somewhere in the middle.
- Mental focus and physical relaxation—meditation and restorative yoga—are two of the most powerful, accessible skill sets to activate recovery.
- If you are breathing deeply and paying attention, you are resting right.
- Distractions are normal—stay with your practice!
- Physical tension often lingers. Your rest space is an opportunity to become aware of how this is manifesting so that you can begin to unwind it.
- So much of what we perceive as more or better energy relates to circulation, and gentle mobility practice supports better flow.

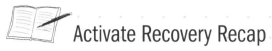

Activate Recovery Recap

Pause and feel the difference.

Has your perception of how to rest and recover shifted at all? How?

What mental practices resonate?

What physical practices resonate?

Have any practices surprised or challenged you? Which and how?

How would you answer this question now, having explored some of the tools for activating real recovery: When you stop, what should you do?

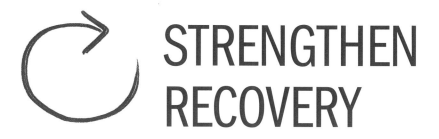

STRENGTHEN RECOVERY

Create Your
Recovery Practice

You've now become more receptive to rest by opening your mind to a restorative approach, and you've explored some practical tools and ways to activate real recovery. Now it's your practice—attention and reps—that is the real game changer. Consistent practice is what will increase your ability to use rest to full advantage and to become more fluent in recovery.

It's time to create your recovery practice. But what is a practice? And how do you create it?

Use this chapter to put rest into practice in your way.

Welcome to Your Practice Meditation

This simple gesture of meeting yourself where you are is a natural entry point to your practice, a settling and restorative inward movement. Notice what it feels like as you connect to yourself in these moments.

- Sit comfortably.
- Take a deep breath in… a slow breath out…
- Continue to deepen your breathing.
- Acknowledge, this is it—you're here now, practicing rest.
- Slow down, breathe deeply, pay attention…
- Feel yourself settling into your practice, into yourself.
- Keep breathing deeply.
- Feel the comfort of knowing this space, your practice, is yours to return to as needed, a baseline that supports you to stay aware of where you are and to respond accordingly.
- Acknowledge this input and keep moving toward recovery.

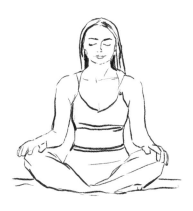

If you are breathing deeply and paying attention, you are resting right.

Your Practice

Practice is something you do habitually and on purpose. Taking a few deep breaths to calm yourself when you're stressed—that's a practice. So is lifting weights to maintain your strength. Taking your kid out on their bike to build their confidence and lose the training wheels—also a practice. Recovery is no different—it's a self-supporting practice that you strengthen with repetition. Practice increases our capacities and strengthens our tolerance for what might have once felt difficult.

Practice connects the dots—it creates balance.

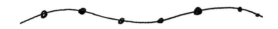

Just as you might strengthen your core to ease back pain, you can begin to solve the macro discrepancy between work and rest, working out and working in, by activating recovery. Once you understand how to activate your core, perhaps with help from a physical therapist, you'll make a plan to use those exercises to strengthen it, and you'll probably consider practicalities like when and where you'll practice. Recovery is no different. Once you understand how to activate your mind and body into a restorative state, it's your repetitive practice that builds equity with recovery and yields the results you seek.

The more you practice, the more you strengthen your practice "muscle." Regardless of your unique approach—you create it and strengthen it by doing it often. Like a muscle, the more you use it, the stronger it becomes. As you feel the difference—the benefits—of your consistent effort, you'll be motivated to practice more and continually reap the benefits.

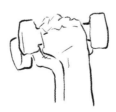

Practice Is Your Baseline

Recovery practice is an ongoing check in with yourself—it establishes a baseline for where you're at and how you're doing. It's an ever-available, internal place where you can recharge and recenter yourself amid life's inevitable uncertainty, change, and imbalance. Your restful pauses disrupt the inertia of daily going, making, and doing and create space for you to slow down, breathe deeply, and pay attention—to be. Just as you might feel relieved or comforted as you return home after a long, busy day, your practice is a space to regroup and renew yourself.

Every time you come to your practice, it's like you're beginning again, a gentle do-over. It's a new prompt and opportunity to pause (really, pause) to check in with yourself, which will bring new insights day to day and moment to moment about how you are and how you might support yourself.

Rest—practice—and start again.

 ## Find Your Baseline

When you come to practice, pause to notice how you feel. Maybe you've already noticed fatigue, and that's motivated you to rest (yes!), or maybe you're stopping for a scheduled break (that's great too!). These observations create a baseline for comparison post-practice and help you to feel the difference, which is a motivating force to keep practicing.

Practice is...

It doesn't have to be formal or fancy. There are so many ways to practice and, in doing so, uphold your well-being. What other notions or words come up for you?

a well-timed pause
meeting yourself where you are

habitual
ritual
repetitive
a little, often

checking in
purposeful
momentary pauses
simple gestures
attention

recalibration
connecting to center
strengthening
progressive
forward movement

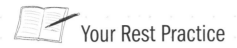

Your Rest Practice

Reflect on what recovery practice means to you.

What restorative practices do you use in your life/work/training?

How do these practices support you?

What motivates you to practice rest?

Your Context

Recovery is incredibly personal and unique to you. Remember, if your practice doesn't fit in your real life, it won't work. For your practice to make an impact, it needs to be contextual, taking into account your goals, circumstances, and practicalities. Ticking the box doesn't really get the job done. Infusing the motions of your practice with your context is the path to longevity and meaningful results.

Context is the factors that align your practice to your circumstances and goals. It informs your practical application of recovery and guides you to discern what to do and how and when to do it. Context frames your knowledge of what you want to work toward (your focus or goal) with your understanding of what needs to be done (your approach) and prompts action (your plan and practice). This knowledge and understanding of what's important to you and what's needed will fuel your motivation to practice and, ultimately, grow in a positive direction. Context is the key!

You're here moving toward ease for a reason. You've heard recovery is important, you're not sleeping well, you're so tired of being tired… whatever sparked your interest in recovery and using this book is a great place to start considering your context as it relates to recovery. Your intention, mission, focus, goal—whatever best describes your own personal north star—drives your approach and your plan. With clarity around why you're here and what context you'd like to prioritize, you can more readily articulate what's needed and create a personal, actionable practice and plan that generates real results.

Pause and revisit your opening notes on your intention for your time with this book (page 9). How might this context inform your practice?

Context powers practice.

Context Is Dynamic

Context is as dynamic as daily life. We all live in many contexts—wear many different hats, play different roles. This is true whether you are an athlete and like to live in a sports context that revolves around the particulars of your training schedule, you're a corporate executive and find yourself immersed in a continual cycle of deliverables and deadlines, you're self-employed and hustling to manage all the moving parts of your work and business, or you're a parent navigating the diverse demands of caring for a family. Chances are you find yourself at an intersection of multiple contexts on a daily basis. Maybe a few different areas came up for you in the preceding prompts? That's okay!

It's useful to acknowledge that we are all holding a lot—and that we all need support. As you practice resting in order to uphold yourself in different areas of your life, you'll become aware of rest's ability to broaden your perspective and capacity, helping you to more fluidly navigate different contexts that come up for you.

Come Back to Context

Checking in with your context is checking in with yourself. Like balance and practice, context is fluid, changing from day to day and even moment to moment. Your rest context—the practicalities that inform what kind of recovery is needed, and when and how it's needed—are likely to shift often.

Maybe you find yourself on a difficult project at work—it's time-consuming, tedious, and even uninspiring and leaves you feeling flat and lethargic. A timely way to respond to this context could be more short bursts of rest, often, leveraging gentle movement to improve circulation and energy for fueling you through a challenging stint.

Or you're rising early to get your workout in before full, busy days. Don't be surprised if you feel a more distinct dip later in the day as a result of those early alarms and sweat sessions, especially when strung together over multiple days. If you're going to rise and run, your rest context might ask you for an earlier bedtime or even an afternoon power nap.

And sometimes, when it all feels like too much, it might help to acknowledge the reality that it is indeed too much and give yourself permission to set it all down, even for a few minutes, and rest. If you're tired, don't give up. Rather than imploding, rest and start again.

Your context will tell you how best to rest, regardless of what's coming at you, and responding to these practicalities in real time will keep you moving forward in a more balanced, sustainable way.

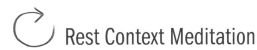

Rest Context Meditation

Every time you come to your practice, check in with your context. These insights help you to realign what is important, what is needed, and how to support yourself.

- Sit comfortably.
- Take a deep breath in… a slow breath out…
- Continue to deepen your breathing.
- Take a moment to consider context—this is what brought you here and makes your practice uniquely relevant to you, makes it yours.
- What context comes forward? This could be a goal that's brought you to practice, an awareness of an imbalance…
- What is your context for your rest practice?
- Notice what comes up, feels timely or relevant, and gently turn your attention toward those priorities to guide your practice.

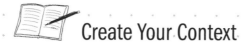

Create Your Context

Consider your context and all its practicalities.

What are your key recovery contexts? What facet of your life do you hope rest will serve?

What are some of the practicalities of that context—how does that inform how you might practice rest?

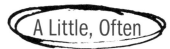

A Little, Often

You know that contextual practice supports your well-being and supercharges your ability to rejuvenate in a meaningful way. Now it's time to think about the practicalities of actually using your practice. While recovery is incredibly complex and dynamic, and also personal to you, it's also really simple. All you have to do to get this going, gain momentum, and feel the difference across whatever contexts are coming up for you is to start now—a little, often.

Don't worry, you don't have to do more or do it better to feel the difference. Doing a little matters, but it's in doing those little bits often enough while paying attention that they become a practice. Remember that it's the power of practice that ultimately makes this work.

So often, we defeat ourselves before we've even started because we don't have a lot of time, our plans have changed, or we're not totally sure what to do in the moment. Maybe you missed a chance to put your legs up the wall because a call came in, or you scrolled social media during your break instead of pausing for the brief meditation you had planned, or just as your run ended you checked your messages rather than stretching your hamstrings. Oops. It's okay! Give yourself a do-over—reset your mindset. There's still time to do what you can, and acknowledging the power in that is a brave thing (see I Don't Have Time, page 24 for more inspiration).

Exhale completely, soften your gaze, use the stretch, slow down for a moment. The briefest gestures often hold the power to bring the biggest results. If you pay attention to the abundance of restful moments available to you—and use them—you'll quickly find that it adds up to a lot, and it all counts. More importantly, you gain equity with rest by experiencing the repetition needed to shift your mindset and behavior to create a practice that works for you.

You don't need a big fancy plan to gain from rest. What matters is that you use your practice to balance your full life with rest in the moments when you need it most.

 ## Lay Down Your To-Dos

After I do x, y, z, I'll finally be able to rest. Sound familiar? This way of thinking implies that we can't rest until everything is done and, let's be honest, there will always be more to do. Every time we say things like this, it strengthens an imbalanced mentality and keeps us running on the wheel of endless action. Get out of your own way by laying down your to-do list, knowing that it will be there, right where you left it... after you rest. With practice, you will learn to trust that you'll be able to attend to your list more effectively after you've recharged.

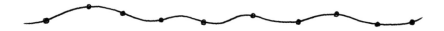

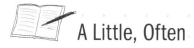

A Little, Often

Think about how a little, often, makes an impact. Be creative—consider what you can do in the time you do have to support yourself, even as schedules shift and the unexpected inevitably arises.

What do you need to do to address the key contexts you've identified?
(Refer back to Create Your Context, page 118.)

How will you integrate recovery into your schedule?

Be realistic—what could your practice look like on a daily or weekly basis?

What are potential challenges to daily practice? Keep it real. What kinds of unforeseen disruption might force you to change your approach or plan in real time?

How can you be fluid in your approach and practice daily, regardless of what comes up? How can you use your practice to create more balance amid the unpredictable nature of daily life?

Keep practice real.

Ebb + Flow

There is a natural ebb and flow as we move through the day. Your energy levels rise and fall, and your mind, body, and nervous system are constantly communicating and responding to what you are doing. You might find that, by nature, you're a lark or a night owl, more energetic earlier or later in the day.

We support ourselves by recognizing and moving with these rhythms, rather than fighting against them. Even your breathing so often reflects the flow of each day's energy and activities. Have you noticed? Inhaling mirrors the uplift and extension of energy required for certain events and activities, while exhaling accompanies the slowing and release that comes when we are on the other side of those outputs. If you pay attention, you can connect to this natural rhythm and use it to full advantage as you move and breathe through your day.

 Pay attention to your inhales and exhales.

Inhale

getting ready for work
reviewing the day's schedule
making coffee
warming up for a workout
important appointments
a challenging conversation
the school run
studying
deep work

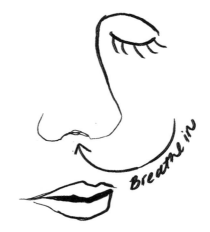

Exhale

lunchtime
a quiet walk
a cup of tea between meetings
heading home from work
putting devices away
tucking kids into bed
restorative stretching
journaling
reading before going to sleep

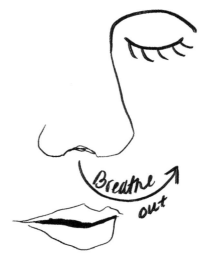

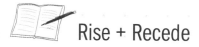

Rise + Recede

Reflect on how your energy ebbs and flows throughout the day. Sketch a line to help visualize what that looks like, along with any notes that feel applicable. For example, you might note an upswing as your day begins, perhaps with a frazzled flurry just before you break for lunch, at which point your energy might dip into a midday or early afternoon valley. Perhaps you have a second wind or burst later in the afternoon?

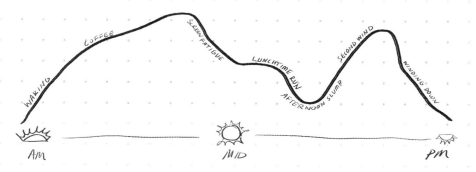

How does your energy typically flow throughout the day?

What activities feel like an inhale and which feel like an exhale?

Notice the points when your energy wanes. How might you better support yourself at those junctures with restorative practice?

Breathe in and breathe out, ebb and flow...

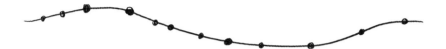

Seasons + Cycles

There are, of course, broader seasons and cycles we navigate throughout life that impact how we feel and how much rest we need at any given time. We're all in a constant state of change, and our ability to rebound from effort shifts as we age. Our longevity depends on how well we adapt to these changes and respond by supporting ourselves where we are.

A more active phase of your career, a challenging training cycle in the lead-up to a key event, or, if you are a woman, where you are in your menstrual cycle or the broader hormonal shifts that accompany the pregnancy and postpartum periods, perimenopause, menopause, and beyond, will all affect how much rest you need, and this should be acknowledged and respected. And naturally, all of these factors will impact your energy and capacities.

Tuning in to the natural world also provides timely inspiration. While summer is a season of expansion—longer, brighter days with an abundance of activity and connection—winter is naturally a slower, more introspective time. The warmer months tend to usher in more energy and capacity for output, while the cooler months invite more rest and reflection. Spending time in nature and paying attention to how seasonal shifts affect our internal rhythms, and responding accordingly, is a powerful, accessible way to support your sense of balance and well-being.

These cycles are natural and needed, and we'd be wise to attune to the natural flow of rest rather than swim against the current. Embrace your seasons and cycles of retreat and expansion, resting and rising. This is a practice in itself.

Respect where you are and your need for rest.

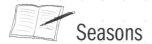 Seasons

Consider what season you're in now and how that impacts your need for rest.

What season is it (winter, spring, summer, autumn) and how is your energy responding to that?

What is needed? How might you support yourself with rest this season? What other cycles impact your need for rest?

Are you training for an event? Where are you in your training cycle, and how does rest best fit in?

If you're a woman, what season are you in hormonally, and how might rest help?

Transitions

It's easy to get caught up in your schedule and the headlines of the day. But what about the space in between? If you pay attention, you might notice that you're leaning forward, pace slightly up-tempo, or even fully rushing. But do you need to be? Sometimes, sure, yes. But more often than not, no. We're so accustomed to a fast pace that we don't even notice how much we're leaning in and how much additional energy we're expending needlessly.

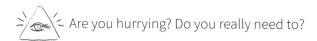 Are you hurrying? Do you really need to?

Something is ending and something is beginning, but without a transition, we end up rushing from one thing to the next without reflecting on or integrating what has happened or preparing for where we're heading. There's a certain residue, a buildup, that accumulates when we operate in this randomized way. Carrying around the wispiness of all these things is tiring!

Look closely and you'll see transitional space everywhere— cooling down from your workout, peeling off for a lunchtime breather, heading to the school pickup… these are underutilized spaces to reset and feel more spacious, allowing you to move through your day with more ease.

For example, one thing I've done as a daily practice since my children reached school age is to create a distinct transition from work to kid pickup. At least 20 minutes before I know I need to be en route, I close my laptop, set a timer for 10 to 15 minutes, and put my legs up the wall. Breathing deeply, I find myself thinking about work yet to be completed and reminding myself to bring snacks, but the thoughts slow and settle after a few minutes, and it feels good to flip my legs upside down after sitting. When I take this time to transition, I'm far more calm and present, available for whatever meets me at the school gate. It's a way that I've been able to better support my family by resting myself.

Use transitions to rest.

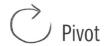 Pivot

Transitions are a natural prompt to end one thing and move toward the next with more ease.

- As you complete a task or activity, pause for a moment.
- Sit comfortably or set yourself up in a restorative posture, such as Legs Up the Wall (page 94) or Child's Pose (page 96), if you have time.
- Take a deep breath in… a slow breath out…
- Continue to deepen your breathing.
- Acknowledge what you've just done or completed. Reflect for a moment on what went well or what didn't, make a few mental notes… If there's more related activity, set a time when you can return to it later, but allow yourself to release it for now.
- Take another deep breath and continue until you feel more settled.
- Consider your next activity or commitment and begin to give that specific thing your attention—not the string of things it could lead to or what you have to do afterward, just focus on what's next.
- Take another deep breath and keep yourself slower, more present, as you pivot toward what's next.

Similarly, after any restorative practice, don't leap into action—don't feel like you instantly have to catch up with everything after you've had a rest. Suspend the calm you've reestablished with a few more deep breaths, resist the urge to check your phone notifications, and take your time moving into the next thing, creating a smoother reentry into the flow of your day. This is how you can be more present and available to whatever comes at you.

Quell Your Adrenaline

If you're just wrapping up a hard workout or intense burst at your desk, use your Pivot practice (page 133) to move back into life with more ease.

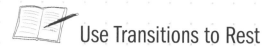

Use Transitions to Rest

Consider the events of your day and then identify the space between activities.

Where are your transitions?

How can you use them to rest and reset, and in doing so ready yourself for what's next?

Daily Anchors

Our most common, universal daily anchors are probably mealtimes. We need food to live, and most of us plan this fuel around a cadence of breakfast, lunch, and dinner. Given that rest is another of the most essential human needs, what if you considered and planned your rest refuels in a similar way? Using rest to frame your day might seem radical, but it shouldn't.

Morning, midday, and evening are natural points of transition throughout your day—spaces between sleeping and waking, coming and going. These are natural prompts to plan and review, to pause, check in, and respond. If we pay attention, we can infuse these moments with rest and, in doing so, more effectively sustain our energy throughout the day, even as we take care of things and navigate the unexpected.

Consider rest as you frame your day.

Use these prompts and practices to help you find a more easeful rhythm each day.

Morning: Align and Set the Tone

Rather than leaping out of bed and springing into action, consider a gentler start and plan accordingly to make that possible for yourself. Notice the difference between easing into your morning and rushing into your to-do list. Even as you breathe into your morning with all its activities, commitments, and possibilities, you have the power to set the tone.

Center Yourself

Use your morning practice to greet yourself gently, establish a steady pace, and set the tone for the day ahead.

- Sit comfortably—center your body front to back, right to left, top to bottom. Keep wiggling around until you feel centered in your seat, then relax into that posture (no need to be rigid about it).
- Take a deep breath in… a slow breath out…
- Continue to deepen your breathing.
- Inhale as you count 1-2-3-4.
- Exhale as you count 1-2-3-4.
- Breathe in for 4…
- And out for 4.
- Continue to even and balance your inhales and exhales as you sit comfortably and centered.

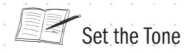 ## Set the Tone

Consider how activating rest could steady you for what each day holds.

How do I want to feel today?

How will rest support that?

What is one practice I'll use to rest and recover?

What's one unexpected spot where a pause might serve me well?

Midday: Check in and Refresh

You might notice there's a point in your day, perhaps late morning as your caffeine fix wears off, after lunch, or post-workout, when there's a distinct slowdown. Your energy wanes, your mind becomes foggy, your body feels stiff. This is usually inconvenient—there's loads left to do. This is when we really benefit from a restorative boost. Rather than reaching for a sugary or caffeinated quick fix that's likely to leave you crashing again before you know it, reach for rest.

 ## Have a Rest Snack

What if you reached for rest when you notice fatigue in the same way you reach for a snack when you're hungry? You can. Try it and feel the difference.

Reach for rest.

↻ Shake It Out

Remember that so much of what we perceive as more or better energy is often better circulation. This is where mobilizing practices (see Recirculate, page 101) can be particularly supportive and rejuvenating.

- Stand up.
- Lift up your right foot and shake it, gradually moving the jiggle through your calf, then into your thigh, and eventually to your glute—shake it all out.
- Switch and shake out your entire left leg.
- Then shake your hands, moving through your wrists and up your forearms, your elbows and upper arms, eventually to your shoulders, then shaking out your whole spine all the way up to your neck.
- Now shake everything—lower body, upper body, head…
- Continue for 30 seconds.
- Come to stillness and breathe deeply.
- Pause and feel the difference.

Wiggle your parts and they will work better.

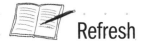 **Refresh**

Think about how you can use rest to sustain you.

What's my usual go-to when my energy wanes?

Does that really recharge me?

What restful gesture might better refuel me to do what I need to do?

Evening: Wind Down and Review

Winding down can be tricky. Remember, we don't go from 60 to 0 by default. After sprinting through the events of the day, it's common to feel like it's all a blur and there isn't much space, especially in your mind. Consciously putting a little bit more space between each one of your thoughts helps to slow things down in your head, supporting you to more easefully transition to a restful evening and, ultimately, a better night's sleep.

 # Wind Down

Use this practice to welcome yourself to your evening, review how you've moved through your day, and release any lingering tension as you transition from work to rest.

- Sit comfortably.
- Take a deep breath in… a slow breath out…
- Continue to deepen your breathing.
- Once your breath feels steady, inhale deeply and hold your breath for a moment, holding only one thought with that breath.
- Exhale slowly, letting that thought go.
- Again, inhale deeply, perhaps with a different thought… hold, then exhale, letting go of that thought and moving on to the next one.
- Continue, with just one thought per breath, creating and feeling more space as you breathe.

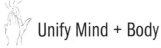 ## Unify Mind + Body

Couple your mental unwind with your favorite restorative posture. If unsure, practice Legs Up the Wall (page 94) or Activate Physical Relaxation (page 91), which encourage a deeper settling and postural reset than flopping onto a couch or your bed.

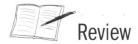 # Review

Take a moment to review the contents of your day.

How did my work/rest balance feel today?

What were the challenges?

What were the wins?

How might I better support myself tomorrow with the rest I need?

Quick Resets

We've covered a lot up to this point. What might be most useful now is to simplify and consolidate your understanding by remembering that rest is readily available. Rest doesn't have to be formal or fancy, and recovery doesn't have to be an official meditation or yoga session. What matters is your practice, and that you continue to pay attention to how you are and respond by doing something—anything—to rest. Acknowledge where you are in the work/rest balance and choose to recharge in the moments when you need it most. Trust that the smallest gestures found in the most ordinary moments can create big containers for rejuvenation when you use them often.

 What do you do when rest feels out of reach?

Remember, if you're breathing deeply and paying attention, you are resting right. Honor the realities of your full life by using these brief practices that can fit seamlessly into the flow of your day.

↻ The 2-Minute Reset

When it comes to recovery, anything is better than nothing. Thirty seconds? Yes! Two minutes? Let's do this. Use rest in the time that you have. While it's great to have an unrushed routine and a distraction-free setting, that's not always practical—and that's okay.

For example, your day might be hectic, but chances are you can still pause, breathe deeply, and settle down in the time it takes your coffee to brew. Or before you show up to that next meeting. Or while you're in the car waiting for your kid.

Recognize those mini pockets of time and own them. Claim them as rest time. The more often you practice, the more readily you'll be able to access the rest that's available right in front of you.

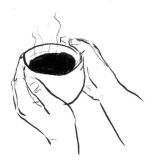

Any rest is better than none.

↻ Feel Your Feet

Pause, close your eyes, and feel where your energy is—notice where it is in your body. If you are busy, multitasking, or stressed, you might notice more sensation, tension, or a buzz in your head, chest, or elsewhere in your upper body. Now focus on your feet and notice how deliberately shifting your focus downward helps you to calm down and feel more grounded. Wiggle your toes, it helps!

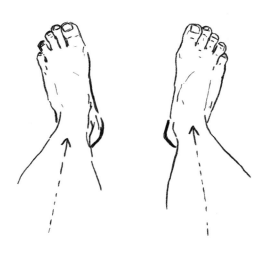

Close Your Eyes

Gently close your eyes to create a distinct shift from out to in, from external stimulation to internal experience—which is where real recovery happens. Linger here for a few moments or set a timer if you like, resting your eyes and allowing yourself to settle down from the inside out.

Move inward.

Horizon Gaze

Let's be honest, we could also call this a technology break. While your focus is usually narrowly focused on the task at hand and anticipating the next thing, pausing to look up and out at the horizon—ideally a green space—can help to recharge your attentional capacity. Even if you're busy at your desk, when you look out the window, your very directed attention shifts to a softer focus—relaxing your mind, relieving tension in your physical structure, encouraging your breathing to expand, and broadening your perspective.

Better yet, place your face in the sun for a few minutes, if you have access, even if through a window—that's a quick way to reset screen fatigue.

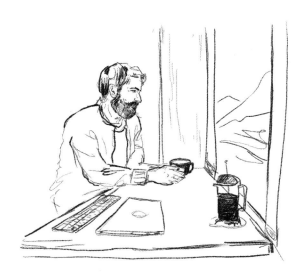

Pull Your Head Off

Consider brain cramps, mental stagnation, or overly feral thoughts a good reset prompt. Use this practice to calm your nervous system, release tension, and reset your foggy and/or busy mind.

- Stand with your feet hip-width apart.
- Fold forward, bending your knees as much as needed to allow your torso to rest close to your thighs.
- Drop your head.
- Interlace your fingers at the back of your neck or the base of your skull.
- Press the sides of your head with your forearms.
- Lengthen toward the floor, as if you're (gently) pulling your head off.
- Stay for 5 to 10 deep breaths.

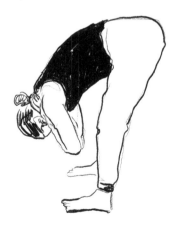

⟳ Forward Fold at the Wall

While not a classic restorative posture, folding forward in this manner is a naturally introspective gesture and an energizing reset. This setup also encourages your spine and hamstrings to lengthen, which is timely when you've been sitting for a prolonged period of time, and leaning back into the wall removes the work of balancing.

- Lean into the wall with your feet hip-width apart and parallel, a foot or two away from the wall.
- Keeping your knees slightly bent, fold forward and walk your hands down your legs.
- Lean back into the wall. If you feel like you can't lean back, bring your feet a bit farther away from the wall.
- Rest your hands wherever they land or on props, if needed.
- Stay for 5 to 10 deep breaths.

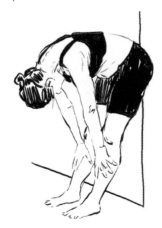

Legs Up the Sofa

Here's another inverted posture ever available in your living room, bedroom, or anywhere you can find a surface about the height of your thigh bones. In this inverted setup, you gain the benefit of recirculating excess blood and fluid in the legs, plus it's an easy way to neutralize your spine and bring more ease to your back.

- Lie down on the floor, bend your knees, and rest your lower legs on a couch, chair, or any surface roughly the height of your thigh bones.
- Rest your arms open, palms up.
- Stay for 5 to 10 deep breaths, or set a timer for 5 to 15 minutes.

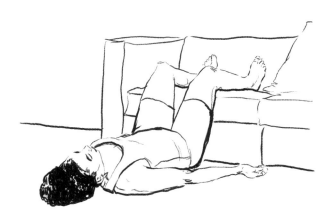

Use Your Rest Power Stance

Of all the different mental and physical approaches and tools for rest we've explored, what's been a quick win for you? What connected—replenished you—efficiently in the moment? Maybe it's extending your exhalations (page 82), pulling your head off (page 151), or putting your legs up the wall (page 94). Note anything that makes a fast, noticeable difference and consider it a restorative power stance that you can turn to without planning, thought, or effort when you feel stressed or short on time.

More, When Needed

While a little, often, is practical and impactful, when feasible it can be useful to carve out more time and space to unwind and recharge—to create a bigger container for recovery. This is likely to seem more available or be prompted by junctures or practicalities such as wrapping up a big project at work, completing a big race or competition, or when your kids have a school break. Look for these natural cues and embrace them as an opportunity to shift gears and recharge.

And sure, it's great to go on a vacation, or maybe you'd love a spa day, but you don't have to get on a plane or lie on a beach, or even have an entire free day, to extend your reset.

For a bigger container for rest, consider creating practical pockets of time:

- Clear your mornings for a few days or a week, and don't set an alarm.
- Say no thank you to weekend plans and wind down your week without an agenda, knowing you have two days ahead to slow down and chill out.
- Decrease your stimulus. Give yourself permission to take a few days (or even a few hours) off from responding to messages and take a break from social media—unplug from your devices.
- Schedule time for yourself to do something you love but rarely have time to engage with, such as hiking, reading a book, lingering in your garden...

Creating these containers is something to be proactive about. Don't wait until you're burned out or in a deep valley of fatigue to consider taking time off. As you consider these resets, you might also become aware of a few missed opportunities. Do your "vacations" feel like hard work? Are your weekends more exhausting than your weekdays? These are prompts to have a closer look at how you're using your precious time off.

Gentle reminder: Rest.

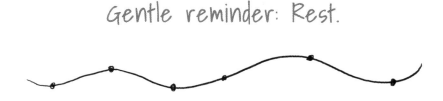

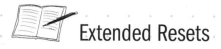

Extended Resets

Reflect on your time off and how you use it to rest and recharge.

What are some things you find yourself doing during days off or vacation time that further drain you?

What are some favorite resets that fit in with your daily practicalities? How can you enjoy more reps, potentially by creating bigger containers for them?

What restorative activities or practices could you leverage when you have extended time?

Rest Recap

You know why recovery matters, and when and how to activate it. Now it's your practice that generates results. Continue to evolve your practice, knowing that it will be as fluid and dynamic as your days. With your attention and reps, you'll gain rest fluency and feel the difference.

- Practice is a game changer.
- Context powers practice.
- A little, often, is powerful approach to real recovery when you use small resets often enough that they become a practice.
- There's a natural ebb and flow to your energy throughout the day, as well as seasons and cycles that will influence how much rest you need.
- Transitions are everywhere—use them to reset.
- Morning, midday, and evening are natural prompts to plan, review, and rest. Consider these anchors as you frame your day.
- Practice doesn't have to be formal or fancy—quick resets can help you to recharge in the moments when you need it most.
- Rest is a power stance—use it!

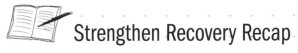

Strengthen Recovery Recap

Pause and feel the difference.

What is restorative practice looking like for you at this point in your journey?

What's the key context for your practice?

What approaches or practices most resonate?

How are you practicing rest?

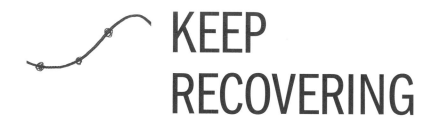

KEEP RECOVERING

Stay with It

At this point, you're further along in your recovery journey than you might realize. Using this book is moving you toward better rest and recovery. Your mindset is becoming more restorative, you're learning powerful, accessible recovery skills, and your rest fluency is improving every time you practice.

Practice

Where to go from here? Your restorative journey is personal. While there is no universal rest prescription that suits everyone, remember that all you need to harness the power of restorative practice is your attention—right now, where you are. Remember also that rest is cyclical; it comes around often, and you need it every day. Just as balance is a constant and ever-evolving adjustment toward center, the rhythm of your rest and recovery will shift and evolve through different seasons and cycles.

Like most aspects of life, the path is rarely linear or predictable. Your restorative practice will continue to swing in the balance, varying from day to day and even moment to moment. Compare today to yesterday, or this week to the same week last month, and you'll see what I mean. Just as balance is a practice, so is recovery. There will be times you feel off course. Consider this recognition an invitation to rest and start again, to reconnect your internal dots so that you can rise to the next challenge.

When you feel unsure, uninspired, or stuck, come back to the simple practice of noticing and responding. Ask yourself:

How am I?

What's needed?

How will I respond?

Keep practicing and you will find a rhythm that feels good to you.

Rest and Recover Every Day

Recovery is complex and dynamic, and it's also really simple: rest and recover every day. Make this your mantra as you meet yourself daily and use this book to plan and review your evolving practice, knowing that your rest needs will be as fluid as your days.

You know that rest is a power stance, and hopefully you've identified a few of its postures that work best for you (see Use Your Rest Power Stance, page 154). These gestures will become more familiar and effective the more you practice. As you gain equity with rest through your reps, you'll become more fluent in resting in ways that truly work for you. You'll be able to more consciously respond to how you are and call the play, day by day.

Practice, like rest, is a rhythm
that shifts from day to day.

Plan

Taking a few moments to proactively plan where to slot rest into your day can be a useful way to activate your restorative mindset, rather than just seeing what happens and hoping for the best. If you wait for the perfect time to rest, it probably won't happen. But if you seed recovery by considering your outputs and how to support yourself with rest before getting swept into the events of the day, you'll be more likely to rest when you can.

As you plan your day and week, consider where recovery fits. If you're able, schedule your rest as you would an important meeting and protect that appointment as if it were nonnegotiable. If you don't immediately see opportunities for rest amid your activities and commitments, come back to a little, often, and create restful pauses in the time you do have. When rest feels impossible, consider that a nudge to rethink what kind of work/rest balance you're creating and living.

Review

As you wind down your day and week, reflect on where recovery fit in, how it helped, and how you might fine-tune your approach and plan to support yourself into a balance that feels better. Take a brief inventory and use the time to consider where rest was available, what felt restful, and how it replenished you.

Notice any patterns in your rest flow and how rest best fits and how you benefit when you practice. Capture insights as you go and know that every restful gesture you make to yourself, however seemingly small, reconnects your internal dots toward balance, increases your resilience, and fuels you to get to where you want to be.

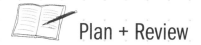

Plan + Review

Use these pages to plan and review your rest daily and/or weekly. You'll find additional Plan + Review pages for you to use to further frame your rest, anchor your wins, and strengthen your recovery practice. Remember that rest shouldn't be another to-do—be fluid in your approach, especially if and when you get caught in the weeds of the day.

How am I?

What's needed?

How will I respond?

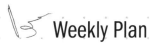 **Weekly Plan**

Key activities/outputs:

Opportunities for rest/inputs (mental and physical):

Ideas for alternative resets if things don't go according to plan:

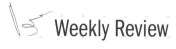# Weekly Review

Recovery wins—when, where, and how I rested well:

How I felt after recovering/the outcome:

Times when I could have chosen a more restorative approach:

How I might fine tune my approach next week:

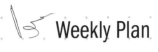 **Weekly Plan**

Key activities/outputs:

Opportunities for rest/inputs (mental and physical):

Ideas for alternative resets if things don't go according to plan:

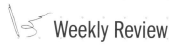 # Weekly Review

Recovery wins—when, where, and how I rested well:

How I felt after recovering/the outcome:

Times when I could have chosen a more restorative approach:

How I might fine tune my approach next week:

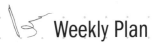 **Weekly Plan**

Key activities/outputs:

Opportunities for rest/inputs (mental and physical):

Ideas for alternative resets if things don't go according to plan:

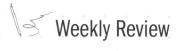
Weekly Review

Recovery wins—when, where, and how I rested well:

How I felt after recovering/the outcome:

Times when I could have chosen a more restorative approach:

How I might fine tune my approach next week:

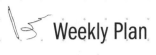

Weekly Plan

KKey activities/outputs:

Opportunities for rest/inputs (mental and physical):

Ideas for alternative resets if things don't go according to plan:

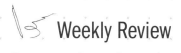 ## Weekly Review

Recovery wins—when, where, and how I rested well:

How I felt after recovering/the outcome:

Times when I could have chosen a more restorative approach:

How I might fine tune my approach next week:

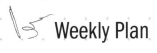

Weekly Plan

Key activities/outputs:

Opportunities for rest/inputs (mental and physical):

Ideas for alternative resets if things don't go according to plan:

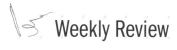 # Weekly Review

Recovery wins—when, where, and how I rested well:

How I felt after recovering/the outcome:

Times when I could have chosen a more restorative approach:

How I might fine tune my approach next week:

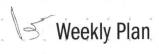 **Weekly Plan**

Key activities/outputs:

Opportunities for rest/inputs (mental and physical):

Ideas for alternative resets if things don't go according to plan:

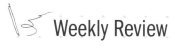

Weekly Review

Recovery wins—when, where, and how I rested well:

How I felt after recovering/the outcome:

Times when I could have chosen a more restorative approach:

How I might fine tune my approach next week:

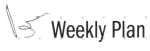 # Weekly Plan

Key activities/outputs:

Opportunities for rest/inputs (mental and physical):

Ideas for alternative resets if things don't go according to plan:

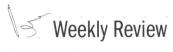# Weekly Review

Recovery wins—when, where, and how I rested well:

How I felt after recovering/the outcome:

Times when I could have chosen a more restorative approach:

How I might fine tune my approach next week:

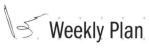 **Weekly Plan**

Key activities/outputs:

Opportunities for rest/inputs (mental and physical):

Ideas for alternative resets if things don't go according to plan:

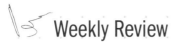# Weekly Review

Recovery wins—when, where, and how I rested well:

How I felt after recovering/the outcome:

Times when I could have chosen a more restorative approach:

How I might fine tune my approach next week:

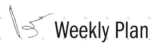 **Weekly Plan**

Key activities/outputs:

Opportunities for rest/inputs (mental and physical):

Ideas for alternative resets if things don't go according to plan:

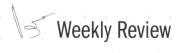 Weekly Review

Recovery wins—when, where, and how I rested well:

How I felt after recovering/the outcome:

Times when I could have chosen a more restorative approach:

How I might fine tune my approach next week:

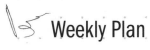

Weekly Plan

Key activities/outputs:

Opportunities for rest/inputs (mental and physical):

Ideas for alternative resets if things don't go according to plan:

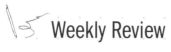 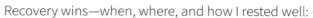

Weekly Review

Recovery wins—when, where, and how I rested well:

How I felt after recovering/the outcome:

Times when I could have chosen a more restorative approach:

How I might fine tune my approach next week:

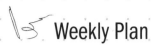 **Weekly Plan**

Key activities/outputs:

Opportunities for rest/inputs (mental and physical):

Ideas for alternative resets if things don't go according to plan:

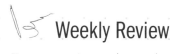 # Weekly Review

Recovery wins—when, where, and how I rested well:

How I felt after recovering/the outcome:

Times when I could have chosen a more restorative approach:

How I might fine tune my approach next week:

Lead by Example

I hope you're feeling the difference at this point on your restorative journey. You're now well equipped to harness recovery's superpowers, not only to support yourself, but to help others, too, because actions speak much louder than words, and your rest impacts everyone around you.

You might have noticed that when you have rested, you're more present and available, maybe even more patient and responsive. Other people feel that. Rest has the power to improve the quality of our interactions and relationships. Not only that, but others are also likely to be inspired and remember their own practice by witnessing yours.

The world pushes us to go, go, go and rarely invites us to stop. Remember, if you don't create space for yourself to rest and model that for your colleagues, teammates, and family, no one else will. Your rest and recovery is your responsibility and your right—make it yours.

Share your rest.

Here are some ways you can lead by example and uplift your community:

- Does your workplace have a room for rest? If not, advocate for a private space where you and your colleagues can go to recharge during your workday—and use it! This type of space has already been implemented by many businesses and is becoming a more standard offering to promote employee wellness.

- Create a rest space at home, perhaps a corner of your bedroom or some other spot where you can calm and center yourself. While you don't really need anything other than your attention, you might choose to set up this area with whatever feels supportive and encourages recovery practice—a yoga mat, some cushions, your journal, and a candle… Invite your family and friends to join you there, sharing your ways of resting. Remember that an open mat can be a powerful visual cue to practice (see Open Your Mat, page 90).

- Does your partner, family, colleague, coach, or team value recovery? If not, share what you've learned and how it's helped you. Be an advocate not just for sporadic rest days, but for intentional daily rejuvenation, and look for ways you can practice this together.

- Protect a more spacious schedule for yourself and your family during weekend or nonworking days. You don't have to fill all the hours or keep up with everyone else.

- Normalize and celebrate rest and recovery by sharing what you do to rest with your people, and ask them how they've been relaxing.

- Share how you are resting on social media and inspire others with **#moverestrecover**.

How can you lead by example? How does your rest benefit everyone around you?

Scan the QR code for exclusive *Move, Rest, Recover* audio and video practices, behind the scenes, guest interviews, and additional resources for your rest and recovery.

For more context and restorative practices, check out *Work IN: The Athlete's Plan for Real Recovery and Winning Results*.

Cheering for you!

Practice Now

Use these pages to locate and move right into timely practices and inspiration in the moments when you need rest the most.

Connect to rest in ways that resonate and work for you.

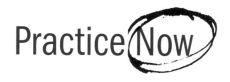

Get out of your own way—rest now.

ACTIVATE RECOVERY— LEARN TO USE REST 57

Mental Focus

Physical Relaxation

STRENGTHEN RECOVERY— CREATE YOUR RECOVERY PRACTICE 107

Practice connects the dots—
it creates balance.

Daily Anchors

Quick Resets

Practice and feel the difference.

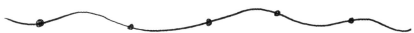

With Thanks

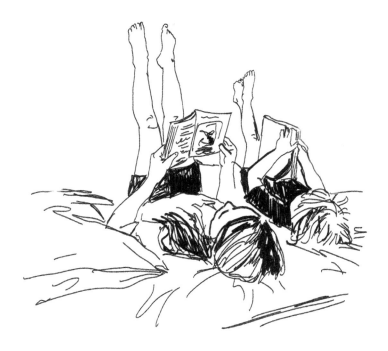

There was a point in this book's creation when I found myself in the convergence of a deadline and no childcare, with work and my young children competing for my attention—a dance many parents know all too well, especially during school breaks. Tension (mine) and silliness (theirs) crescendoed one particular afternoon as I tried to sit with my laptop, and I eventually asked them to go up to their bedroom and calm their bodies down.

I assumed I'd have to intervene further to facilitate their wind down, but within a few minutes all I could hear was the sound of my own typing. I looked up half an hour later and could feel that the energy in the house had shifted completely to a distinct restfulness even as I wrote in haste.

Following my curiosity to see what everyone was up to, I approached their door and heard the sound of pages turning. And there rested my spirited 6- and 8-year-olds, side by side with their legs up the wall, reading books. This scene and their actions served as an affirmation of the very thing I had been writing about:

Rest benefits all of us.

I've spent a lot of time, probably more than most, with my legs up the wall in whatever time I have. It is a practice that evolved over time… during my kids' naps when they were babies, surrounded by toys and a soundtrack of cartoons through the toddler years, and more recently in the evening when we read together. But before this moment I'd rarely seen them use my favorite restorative posture on their own.

Rest is often absorbed in ways that we don't see right away, and not just in ourselves but also in those around us. So often we need to be reminded why, when, and how to rest, and I'm thankful to those who show me this and also reflect the importance of my own actions back to me. Recovery, as it turns out, isn't such a solitary endeavor.

With thanks to the many teachers I've learned and practiced the art and science of rest with—in particular, a deep bow to Elena Brower and Richelle Ricard, two of my dearest, for ongoing support and inspiration.

With thanks to Kierra Sondereker at Ulysses Press, for championing this project and to my longtime editor Renee Jardine, for her ever thoughtful guidance and for always asking the right questions to lead me to my own answers.

With thanks to artist Rebekah MacKay, who has so beautifully brought the ideas and concepts in these pages to life with her eyes, hands, and heart.

With thanks to Rose Sierra and Theo Xander, who continually reframe rest for me in all the best and most important ways.

With thanks to the person who holds me buoyant every day, in all the ways—Mark Taylor.

With thanks to this community near and far—friends, colleagues, and students on the mat with me locally and online worldwide.

And to you, dear reader. Thank you for being here and for valuing your rest and recovery. I wrote this book for you. Remember that when you rest, it serves all of us.

I hope you rest and feel the difference, in your way, every day.

Well done.

About the Author

Erin Taylor is an international recovery expert, writer, and yoga teacher. For 20 years she has coached professional athletes, everyday runners, pre- and post-natal women, office workers, and anyone looking to integrate practices that improve well-being and longevity. She is the creator of *Balance Practice*, a platform that offers practical tools to inspire and support mental and physical balance in all aspects of life. Erin is also the founder of Athletes for Yoga, the only athlete-led, on-demand video platform and app that puts yoga into the context of sport and well-being goals, and the author of *Work IN* and *Hit Reset*.

Learn more and practice with Erin at erintaylor.works.

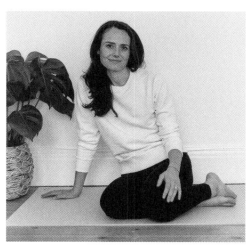

Photograph by Claire Pepper